D1168927

HEALING PSORIASIS:
The Natural Alternative

"Dr. Pagano's book, *HEALING PSORIASIS: The Natural Alternative*, firmly convinces me that he has achieved a phenomenal success in the healing arts—a humane accomplishment. I think it merits world attention. How many poor souls must be waiting in the wings for such a blessed, humanitarian gift!"

PETER HENDERSON, Ed.D.
Author / Journalist / Educator
Haworth, New Jersey

HEALING PSORIASIS

The Natural Alternative

by Dr. John O.A. Pagano
CHIROPRACTIC PHYSICIAN

FOREWORD BY
HARRY K. PANJWANI, M.D., Ph.D.

Also included: A special chapter on ECZEMA

Published by
The Pagano Organization, Inc.
P.O. Box 1215
Englewood Cliffs, N.J. 07632

HEALING PSORIASIS: *The Natural Alternative*

By Dr. John O.A. Pagano
Chiropractic Physician

Published by: The Pagano Organization, Inc.
    P.O. Box 1215
    Englewood Cliffs, New Jersey 07632

DISCLAIMER: The reader should view the material contained herein as a report on the results obtained with patients, based on the research the author has conducted on psoriasis. This information should not be regarded as a guide for self-diagnosis or self-treatment. Consultation with your personal physician prior to embarking on any therapeutic regimen is an absolute necessity.

Library of Congress Cataloging-in-Publication Data:

Pagano, John O.A.

HEALING PSORIASIS: The Natural Alternative

Bibliography   Includes Subject Matter by Chapter

1. Psoriasis   2. Skin Diseases   3. Cayce, Edgar
4. Holistic Medicine   5. Natural Healing

I. Title

CIP 90-92342

ISBN 0-9628847-0-7: $19.95 Softcover

DEDICATION

To my devoted parents,

NETTIE and JOHN J. PAGANO

My beautiful sisters,

CAROL and MARIA

and

SHANE

ABOUT THE AUTHOR

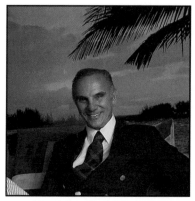

Dr. John O.A. Pagano

Dr. John O.A. Pagano is a graduate of The Lincoln Chiropractic College (now The National College of Chiropractic, Lombard, IL). After serving four years in the United States Navy aboard the Aircraft Carrier "Tarawa" during the Korean War, he entered the School of Visual Arts in New York with aspirations of becoming a medical illustrator. He was torn between art and medicine, so he took courses in both. This training proved invaluable for drawings he made for this book, all of the patient's photography, as well as the cover design. With two years of pre-med and art courses behind him, his interest shifted to the field of chiropractic and he enrolled in The Lincoln Chiropractic College, Indianapolis, Indiana. Upon graduating with honors in 1958, he served his internship at The Spears Chiropractic Hospital in Denver, Colorado. It was during this period that he saw his first psoriasis patient. The impact of viewing this first severe case never left him. Since then, he has relentlessly sought answers to this dermatological enigma.

It was his investigations into the works of the late Edgar Cayce (1877-1945) that provided the clue that set him off on a research project that virtually dominated the major part of his professional career—a span of thirty years. As successful cases continued to mount by following the suggestions made by Cayce, his reputation slowly grew until patient after patient began to seek his help and learn of this new approach to the disease—one free of drugs, tar baths or even ultraviolet light. He only accepted patients that were referred to him by medical doctors, chiropractors, other licensed health practitioners or those who came to him as a last resort having failed to respond to orthodox management. It is because of the results he has achieved, through practical clinical experience, that he now feels he has something to offer the troubled victims of the disease.

Various organizations have requested him to speak in different parts of the country. He has appeared as a featured guest on radio (WABC) and cable TV programs in the New York area and addressed such groups as Bell Laboratories, Hofstra University, William Paterson College and the Parapsychology Society of the United Nations. In November of 1989, he journeyed to India and presented his scientific paper on psoriasis before a body of International Physicians, headed by H.H. The Dalai Lama. In the spring of 1991, he appeared on the popular NBC Television Program, "Unsolved Mysteries."

Now, after fifteen years of concentrated research and eight years of writing, Dr. Pagano's book, *HEALING PSORIASIS: The Natural Alternative*, reveals for the first time in it's entirety, the source of his inspiration, the approach he has taken, and the results he has attained.

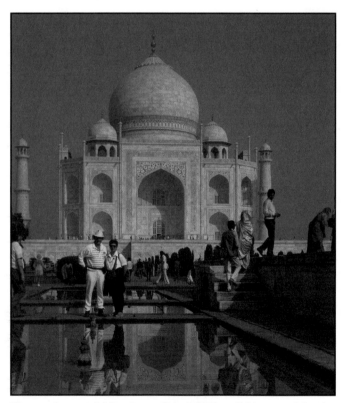

The author and his sister, Carol Miller, R.N., stand in the foreground of the Taj Mahal following a lecture he gave in India on the natural healing of Psoriasis.

Design and Typesetting
by
Typographic Images, Inc.
New York City, New York

Printing and Binding
by
Clarkwood Corporation
Totowa, New Jersey

Cover design: John O.A. Pagano
Cover calligraphy: Jerry Ruotolo

CONTENTS

FOREWORD

The concept of this rather unique and unusual book is to emphasize the power of the human organism to heal the body, with the help of proper diet, posture and gait, attitude and internal cleansing, thus removing the toxins that cause diseases. The regimen outlined in this book pertains to psoriasis—a devastating, humiliating skin disease, usually chronic and recurrent in nature, often leading to depression, despair, other health problems, isolation, and certainly to interference with the sufferer's personal and family life as well as employment and enjoyment of life in general.

There are many references to dietary restrictions for health in the Old Testament. The use of herbs in food or drink is a common practice in Eastern countries like India, China and Japan. For centuries, internal cleansing such as fasting and other methods have been a common practice in European spas to remove toxins from the body. External cleansing is also important, considering the elements to which our skin is exposed throughout the day, in addition to the psychological and cosmetic importance of clean skin.

We, of course, must pay attention to habits and lifestyle, sleep patterns, our environment, and our emotions. The biomechanics of the body—posture and gait—are very important. We have learned in recent years that alternate approaches to health care are being successfully utilized in treating cancer, diabetes, coronary artery disease, stroke, arthritis, depression, and other diseases.

It is essential to ascertain the safety of any treatment and not to overlook other known methods of treatment. This certainly applies to the treatment of psoriasis outlined in this book. In addition to the physical and emotional requirements, we need the open mindedness, the personal sense of morality and spiritual outlook to round off the total approach.

Biofeedback has been in use for many years. It confirms that we can effect biochemical changes in our body when necessary. We need to assume responsibility for our individual health while also recognizing our capacity for self-healing.

Some readers may have difficulty accepting the manner in which Edgar Cayce divined information regarding various health problems. I would like to emphasize that the source of all knowledge or expertise in our life is God, who uses many people as vehicles to make this knowledge or expertise available to others—be they surgeons, pilots, gardeners, teachers or parents. I wholeheartedly recommend this book to the psoriatic or his family, to health professionals and other interested parties for the information it offers.

Harry K. Panjwani, M.D., Ph.D.
Ridgewood, New Jersey

PREFACE

The purpose of this volume is to bring a ray of hope to the tens of millions of people, worldwide, who suffer from psoriasis, one of mankind's oldest, most elusive, chronic inflammatory skin diseases. That hope is not based merely on theory and speculation, but on solid, concrete evidence of results obtained by following a regimen of therapy I have developed over the major part of my professional career—a span of thirty years.

During this period of time, particularly in the past fifteen years, I have concentrated my efforts on proving, indisputably, that psoriasis, long classified as "incurable" by the scientific community, can be healed in a perfectly natural way. The method I have developed is devoid of any drug (systemic or topical, that often have harmful side-effects), uncomfortable "messy" tar baths, or even potentially dangerous forms of ultraviolet light. In short, I contend that psoriasis is one "incurable" disease that the patient does not necessarily have to live with; that it is possible, in many cases, to have every lesion, rash or abrasion of the skin due to psoriasis, disappear completely and leave the patient in control of the problem throughout their entire life. That is the message this book brings forth and is the purpose for which it was written.

It may come as a surprise to many of my readers that I, a chiropractic physician, have taken it upon myself to investigate this dermatological enigma that has frustrated researchers for centuries in seeking a cause and cure. It may come as even more of a surprise to know that the results I have obtained were achieved by practicing well-known, time-honored principles and techniques that fall completely under the heading of natural or holistic healing. In other words, I am utilizing natural methods, in a new way, on an old disease.

It is not my intention to minimize, in any way, the efforts of dedicated researchers and physicians in the field of dermatology. Clearly, they have made life more bearable for many victims of the disease through endless research and various therapies they have developed. Rather, it is my desire to share with them the results I have obtained by revealing the methods I used when attacking this disease from a different perspective—from the inside-out, rather than from the outside-in. Furthermore, the reasons behind every measure in taking this new approach are clearly explained.

Since the cause and true cure for psoriasis remains an "unknown" in the field of dermatology, I ask merely that these findings be taken into consideration. Without question, further research is needed under better controlled conditions, but given the facts contained herein, perhaps a new beginning emerges in understanding the disease which will justify such research. I submit that the information presented herewith warrants such investigation.

The approach to psoriasis that I have used is based on the works of the late Edgar Cayce (1877-1945); a most remarkable individual whose discourses on healing are legendary and are becoming more popular with each passing year. Using his advanced theory as a guide to understanding the cause of the disease, as well as a suggested regimen of therapy, I have combined my clinical experience and slowly evolved a working hypothesis, a natural alternative, that over the years has proven to be extremely beneficial in many cases. It has shown that when psoriasis is understood from this new perspective, faith in the process is strengthened by logic and reason—or, to state it more succinctly, "It makes sense!" in the words of the patients themselves.

Unquestionably, there have been failures as there are in all research projects. However, in practically every case, the reason for failing was found to be the patient's own impatience! Outstanding results were not achieved overnight. Most everyone who succeeded in ridding themselves of psoriasis did so with a great deal of time, honest effort and, above all, *persistence*. Without these invaluable mental ingredients, healing is not only difficult, it is impossible! Unless a patient is *committed* to freeing his or her self of this disfiguring disease, the efforts on the part of both patient and physician ends in futility. It does not necessarily follow, however, that success is guaranteed, but with dedication to the regimen, the chances are infinitely greater. Even to this day when success is achieved, I am no less than amazed to see how a patient's skin can renew itself totally and completely without even a trace of the devastating lesions that once covered the entire body. I believe it can be done for the simple reason that—*it has been done*! This is more than an assumption—it is a declaration, the proof of which is found in the pages that follow.

The late Gina Cerminara, Ph.D., author and lecturer, once told me, quite aptly, that "the secret of good writing is to be understood." For this reason, I have endeavored to *keep it simple* in order for my readers to grasp the underlying principles that will allow them to understand the nature of the disease. Consequently, sophisticated medical terminology was purposefully kept at a minimum. Hopefully, I have succeeded.

I look upon this research as a modest beginning in understanding the nature of the disease. Although there are still questions to be answered, the veil of secrecy is slowly being lifted.

Within the pages of this book, psoriasis may be understood for what it is, and with this understanding comes the hope that, despite present conditions, a natural healing is possible. It is my ardent wish that this be so, for then psoriasis sufferers can begin putting their lives in order and get on with this business of living—no longer burdened under the yoke of this disfiguring, all-consuming disease.

January 16, 1991

Dr. John O.A. Pagano
Englewood Cliffs, NJ

NOTE TO MY READERS

"When a thing is understood,
the cure is half accomplished."

Anne Shannon Monroe

PSORIASIS: The "Inside" Story

"Doctor, you must help me—I can no longer go on living this way."

These were the first words Mr. A. uttered to me as I greeted him at my door. He was a friendly, congenial man in his late sixties. Judging by his outward appearance, one would assume there wasn't a thing wrong with him. But something was indeed wrong—radically wrong! When Mr. A. disrobed, I saw the reason for his torment. He was a victim of one of mankind's oldest skin diseases, PSORIASIS.

He had been suffering with the disease for thirty years. It had finally reached a point where over eighty percent of his body was covered with thickened, silvery scales causing pain, bleeding and intolerable itching.

He had heard about me from a local health food store owner who told him that I had helped several psoriasis sufferers. Having exhausted all other available means of fighting the disease, he turned to me in the hope that I might solve his problem.

His case was so severe that I hesitated to accept him as a patient for fear of giving him false hope, even though I had already cleared up a number of similar cases. I had no choice, however, when he pleaded, "Doctor, I have no one else to turn to."

I am happy that he persuaded me to accept him as a patient, for he proved to be totally cooperative. He followed my instructions to the letter, and much to my and his surprise *he was totally clear of all lesions in thirty days!*

This patient was, and still is, the fastest responding case I have ever witnessed. Most patients take from three to six months to show results. Years later, he appeared before a group of my patients to verify his successful recovery. He was an inspiration to all who met him.

His success had come about by following a regimen of therapy based upon a theory never before recognized or even seriously considered by the scientific community. This theory accounts for the success of his and many others whom I had the privilege of treating.

The Cause of Psoriasis

Looking to the skin for the cause of psoriasis is like looking at the tip of an iceberg and assuming it to be the entire structure. One can keep chipping away at the tip, but the iceberg will never disappear. Why? Because its main body lies hidden beneath the surface, and as long as it remains hidden it will continue to exist.

So it is with psoriasis. What one sees on the outside is the physical evidence of something happening *inside* the body. One can treat the outside, but the disease will keep coming back again and again, month after month, year after year, until the patient has exhausted all available avenues of relief. Whom does he turn to? Is there really a remedy to this irritating, often devastating, chronic skin disease? Is it possible for a victim to be free from a lifetime of pain, disfigurement and considerable expense?

The answer to the questions above is an unequivocal YES! There *are* answers to the riddle of psoriasis, answers that have guided me in an effective management of the disease in a safe, natural way.

If a researcher turns to orthodox medicine for an explanation of the cause of this disease, he will still be met today with the same age-old declaration that "there is no known cause or cure for psoriasis." Only an inner belief that there *must* be an answer, although presently unknown, will motivate him to continually seek a solution.

I have done just that by turning to the works of Edgar Cayce, where I found what sounded like a logical explanation for the disease. *"There is a cure...,"*[1] declared Cayce. He then went on to cite the cause and suggest a remedy. The question remained, however, could his theories be proven? This led me into concentrated research covering a period of fifteen years. In that span of time I convinced my patients, as well as myself, that the information provided by the late Edgar Cayce was indeed valid and worthy of serious consideration in the treatment and management of the disease.

In this book, Cayce's information and the concepts drawn from it are revealed as clearly and as simply as possible. Simple, however, does not necessarily mean easy. It all depends on the attitude of the patient. What is easy for one may be looked upon as monumentally difficult by another. I advise my patients to approach the problem in a relaxed, confident way. Anxiety is *not* part of the regimen!

One of my patients cleared up in fourteen months after suffering with psoriasis for fourteen years. He expressed his gratitude when he said, "Fourteen months after fourteen years is not bad." At present (1990), eight years after clearing, he remains satisfied with his results.

Another patient, after staying on the regimen for two weeks, complained "Had I known it was this difficult, I would have never started." Needless to say, she remains a victim of psoriasis.

First, the patient must understand psoriasis for what it is; second, it is important to get on the right track in order to rid oneself of the disease; and third, the patient must have PATIENCE and PERSISTENCE!

The Origin of Psoriasis

As mentioned earlier, to understand the reason for the outward manifestations of psoriasis, one must go inside the body to find the origin. According to the theories advanced by Cayce, that origin is to be found in THE INTESTINAL TRACT. Here is where psoriasis begins, and until this fact is fully grasped and therapy is based on this premise, I believe with utmost certainty that the condition will persist.

What takes place is that the walls in certain areas of the intestinal tract become thin and porous. When this occurs, toxic substances that should normally pass through the intestines and eventually be eliminated by the body, seep through these walls, enter the lymphatic system and invade the blood stream. The body's natural purification system, primarily the liver and kidneys, then tries to filter out these toxins which are building up in the blood. It may take some time, but sooner or later the accumulation of toxins will prove to be more than these organs can effectively handle. When this point is reached, the body's secondary or backup purification systems join in attempting to aid in the process of elimination. When the liver, the major filtering gland of the body, is overloaded, *the skin* comes to the rescue and helps to eliminate toxins. When the kidneys

3

are overtaxed, the lungs come into play. This concept is clearly explained in the works of Henry Bieler, M.D., and is discussed in a later chapter.

A Brief Anatomy Lesson

The digestive tract, the area primarily involved in the origin of psoriasis, is actually a hollow tube with twists and turns throughout the small intestines, carrying out various functions all along its course, from the ingestion of food to the elimination of waste products.

NORMAL DIGESTIVE TRACT:

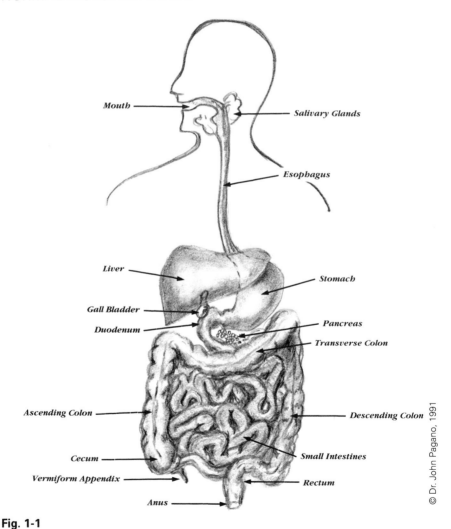

Mouth

Salivary Glands

Esophagus

Liver

Stomach

Gall Bladder

Duodenum

Pancreas

Transverse Colon

Ascending Colon

Descending Colon

Cecum

Small Intestines

Vermiform Appendix

Rectum

Anus

© Dr. John Pagano, 1991

Fig. 1-1

4

When food enters the mouth certain enzymes begin the process of breaking it down for eventual absorption and assimilation in the small intestine. Before food reaches the small intestine, it must pass down a long hollow tube called the esophagus and enter the stomach. There it may remain for hours, being acted upon by more enzymes and certain acids before passing into the first portion of the small intestine, the Duodenum, which is only about 12 inches long. It then enters the next portion of the small intestine, called the Jejunum, which in turn, leads into the Ileum. *It is within these areas, especially where the duodenum meets the jejunum, that the walls of the intestines in the psoriatic become thin and smooth, allowing a transfer of toxins to take place.*[2]

WHERE PSORIASIS BEGINS:

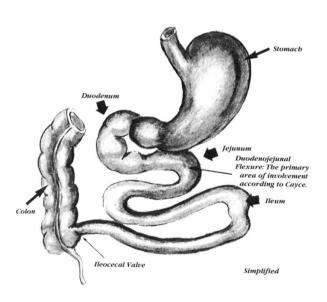

Fig. 1-2

The food, known as chyme at this stage of digestion, continues to move into the Ilium, the longest portion of the approximately 23 foot long small intestine, where nutrients are absorbed and waste matter is passed into the large intestine, the colon, and eventually eliminated.

The FOLDS Throughout the Intestinal Tract

The walls throughout most of the intestinal tract should have certain folds present *at all times,* aiding in the absorption and movement of the contents that are passing through. These folds begin at the latter half of the Duodenum, continue throughout the Jejunum, and end about halfway into the Ileum. They are more concentrated at the *Duodenojejunal Flexure.* (See Fig. 1-2.)

According to the information supplied by Cayce, these are the folds, illustrated below, that become smooth, as though they were thinned out in the psoriatic, permitting a "seepage" of toxins through the walls and eventually into the blood stream. Anatomically, they are called the Plicae Circulares (valves of Kerckring).

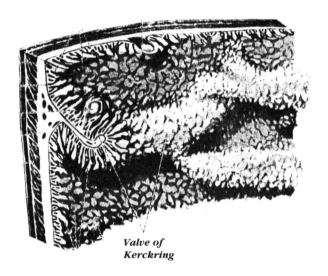

Valve of Kerckring

Fig. 1-3.
Portion of the small intestine; drawn from selections using a binocular microscope. x17. (After Braus.)

Illustration reproduced through the courtesy of the W.B. Saunders Company, Philadelphia, PA. From: *Textbook of Histology,* ed. 10, by Bloom and Fawcett, Copyright 1975, page. 659.

Although the transfer of toxins occurs primarily at the duodenojejunal flexure, this seepage of poisons can and probably does take place throughout the length of both the small and large intestines of a person suffering from psoriasis. The idea, therefore, in this new approach to the disease, is to cut down or preferably stop ingesting pollutants and to strengthen these porous intestinal walls.

Why The Intestinal Walls Become Thin

In his 1968 treatise for the Medical Research Division of the Edgar Cayce Foundation, Frederick D. Lansford Jr., M.D., reports that the smoothing of the intestinal walls does not always have the same cause, but more often than not is due to *improper coordination in the eliminating systems.*[3]

If it is true that the intestinal walls contribute to the development of psoriasis, the next logical question is *why* these walls are thin and porous. The following reasons stand out as the primary factors:

1. Poor elimination

2. Improper diet

3. Misaligned vertebrae

4. Insufficient daily intake of water

5. Negative emotions

6. Hereditary factors

Each of the above will be dealt with as we proceed. Doubtless, some of these conditions overlap each other, contributing to a toxic buildup and causing an increase of *acids* in the blood, which should always be *alkaline.*[4] Therefore, the acid content of the blood must be reduced. Therein lies the basis for the therapeutic regimen outlined in the subsequent chapters of this book.

The "toxic build-up" I refer to is caused not only by those elements that have already been identified as having a poisonous effect on the body, such as carbon monoxide, nitrogen oxides, hydrocarbons, cyclamates and many others. There are substances which are more common but less suspect, especially certain foods, that do not necessarily affect the average person but do indeed play havoc with the psoriatic. They act as allergens to psoriasis victims and turn their life into a living hell. The control of the disease, therefore, is attained primarily by learning to identify those foods that cause a toxic over-acidic reaction in the body and by making it a priority to avoid them at all costs.

Until this concept is fully understood, the patient fights a losing battle. External applications in the form of salves, creams, even ultraviolet light do help in many cases to clear the skin, but they are palliative at best, and before long the condition usually returns, often worse than before. To those relatively few patients who have experienced a spontaneous remission of the disease without ever having a return of symptoms, I say they should thank their lucky stars. For reasons that may never be known, these fortunate individuals were relieved of a lifetime of anxiety and pain.

To those less fortunate, however, I say: TAKE HEART! All is not lost. There is a way out of your dilemma—a natural one that has been proven to be successful in many, many cases.

It is a joy to my patients, as well as to me, to share the knowledge of this alternative path with you in the pages that follow.

REFERENCES

(Chapter 1—PSORIASIS: The "Inside" Story)

1. Edgar Cayce Reference # 2455-2, (Virginia Beach, VA, The Edgar Cayce Foundation, copyright 1971)
2. Ibid # 3373-1
3. Frederick D. Lansford, M.D., "Commentary on Psoriasis" in *Physician's Reference Notebook*, ed. by William A. McGarey, M.D. (Virginia Beach, VA, The A.R.E. Press, Sept. 1968 Ed. 1) p. 189—Extracted from References # 5016-1 and # 622-1.
4. Israel S. Kleiner, Ph.D., *Human Biochemistry*, (St. Louis, The C.V. Mosby Co., copyright 1954, ed. 4) p. 543.

Chapter 2

Does It Work?

My interest in psoriasis actually began while I was an intern in Denver, Colorado. The first case I saw, Mr. D.H., was a pleasant, enthusiastic dairy farmer from southern New Jersey. Since we were from the same state, a friendship as well as a doctor/patient relationship evolved. Although little could be done for his condition at that time, he came every year to the hospital in Denver to take advantage of the bright, sunlit days of Colorado. He said it always helped to clear his skin, if only temporarily. His twenty year battle with psoriasis touched me so deeply that I took a keen interest in learning all I could about the disease. Little did I realize that fifteen years would pass before I met Mr. D.H. again at his home in New Jersey where I showed him the successful results I had attained on my early cases.

In the interim, I kept gathering any information I could on psoriasis. Nothing seemed to hold much promise until I investigated the files on the disease available to me as a member of the Edgar Cayce Foundation in Virginia Beach, Virginia. [*NOTE*: The Edgar Cayce Foundation is the sister organization of the Association for Research and Enlightenment (A.R.E.), headquarters for the Cayce material, located at 67th and Atlantic Ave., Virginia Beach, VA. The numerous files are made available to serious researchers, the over 100,000 members, as well as the general public.]

I carefully studied the two volumes on psoriasis in the circulating files and proceeded to condense the information into a practical working order. Why not, I thought. Since orthodox medicine was still groping for answers, the question remained open. As so aptly stated by Norman Cousins, author of the national best seller *Anatomy of an Illness*, "...the art of healing is still a frontier profession." I proceeded to break down the information and convert it into a practical application. No sooner had I formulated a working hypothesis when my first psoriasis case walked in.

Actually, Mr. William Culmone came to me because of a spinal problem, not psoriasis. [NOTE: Special permission has been granted to use Mr. Culmone's full name.] When he disrobed for his initial examination, my first reaction, although silent, was, "I don't believe this!" Here was an unmistakable, rather severe case of psoriasis. I decided I would only record the fact rather than discuss it with a new patient at our first meeting. My efforts were concentrated on his spinal problem which gradually subsided and disappeared. During each visit I touched upon my studies in psoriasis and my source of information and slowly aroused his interest. By the time his back problem cleared up, he was ready to join me in an experiment, using this new approach to healing psoriasis.

He had tried just about everything else for over fifteen years without results. His was a typical case of common psoriasis with bleeding, itching, scaling and all that accompanies this form of the disease. On July 21, 1975, we began the regimen with the full cooperation of his wife, Minnie. With specific instructions in his possession, he left the office to return in one week.

He came back at the appointed time, disrobed in the examining room and showed me his lesions. I was astonished at the results, for they were at least fifty percent improved. Obviously, a healing was taking place. The large lesion on his right thigh, and several on the lumbar area of his spine were now a light pink color with no scales. They were a far cry from the bloody, crusty patches of seven days earlier.

It took about three months, but on October 16, 1975, Mr. Culmone was no longer a victim of psoriasis. All lesions had disappeared as completely as if someone had used an eraser on his back.

He agreed to put the records of his case on display at the Edgar Cayce Foundation Library in Virginia Beach, hoping that psoriasis victims who saw them would consider following the regimen I had worked out from the information supplied in the Cayce material. Exhibited with his case history and photographs in a special glass display at the library (along with those of several other patients of mine) is Mr. Culmone's signed affi-davit, which reads:

To Whom It May Concern:

RE: Psoriasis Report

This is to verify that the photographs presented in this report, as well as the sequence in which they were taken, were in fact taken at the spec-ified intervals reported herein at the office of Dr. John O.A. Pagano.

The psoriasis I have suffered with for the past fifteen years has virtu-ally "cleared up" in a period of three months from the start of treatment, July 21, 1975. Now (January 15, 1976) I can honestly state that there has been no recurrence whatsoever.

(Signed)
William Culmone

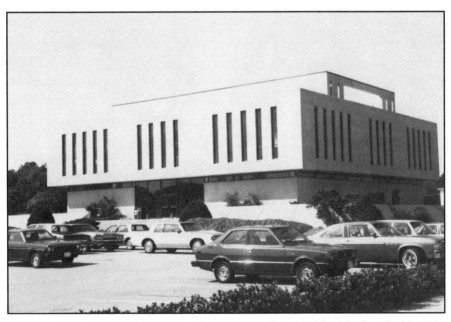

The beautiful A.R.E./E.C.F. Library on the oceanfront in Virginia Beach, Virginia, where the 14,256 discourses (Medical & Non-Medical) are indexed and housed.

Patient: William Culmone
Age: 65 years
Afflicted: 15 years

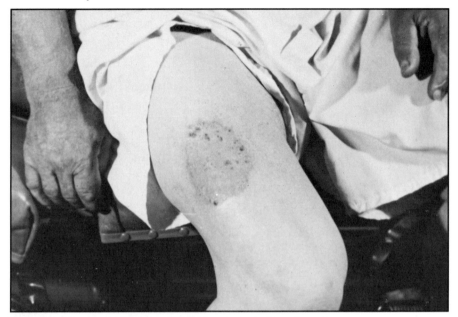

Fig. 2-1 Above photo taken 7/25/75—at start of treatment.

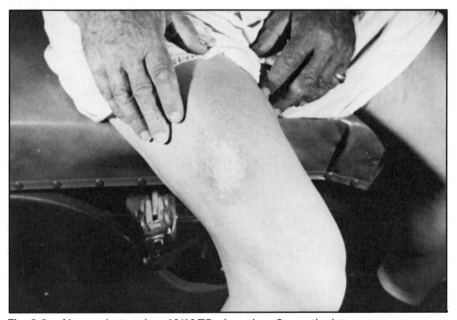

Fig. 2-2 Above photo taken 10/16/75—less than 3 months later.

Patient: William Culmone

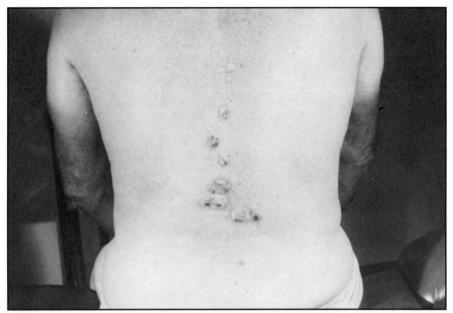

Fig. 2-3   Above photo taken 7/25/75—at start of treatment.

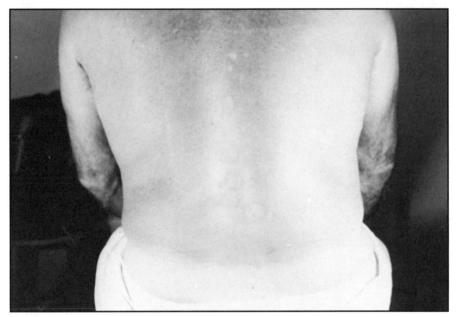

Fig. 2-4   Above photo taken 10/16/75—less than 3 months later.

Mr. Culmone remained clear of all lesions for the remainder of his life. He died years later of unrelated causes. He will always remain in my memory as the first patient who was healed of psoriasis by following this new, natural approach to healing the disease. Mr. Culmone contributed much to all psoriasis victims by his unselfish attitude and willingness to discipline himself.

This first healing set the stage for all my future cases, yet many years passed before I was truly convinced that this was the basic procedure to follow in clearing psoriasis.

My next severe case was that of Mrs. B.K., who took four months to clear up; then a little boy, A.S., who also responded beautifully in four months; then a little girl, E.L., who took about three months. Others followed in rapid succession. The die was cast, my destiny set. I knew I had to continue with my research until it culminated in incontrovertible evidence that this approach did indeed heal psoriasis.

The Early Cases

PERMISSION HAS BEEN GRANTED BY EACH PATIENT TO USE THE PHOTOGRAPHS THAT FOLLOW FOR THE PURPOSE OF THIS REPORT. INITIALS HAVE BEEN USED TO PROTECT EACH PATIENT'S RIGHT TO PRIVACY.

Patient: B.K.
Age: 32
Afflicted: 2 years

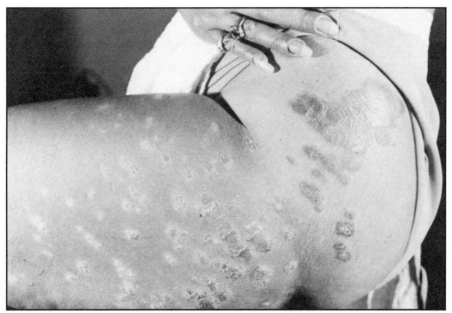

Fig. 2-5   Above photo taken 9/3/76—at start of treatment.

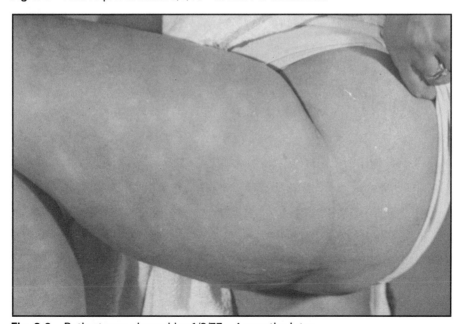

Fig. 2-6   Patient was cleared by 1/3/77—4 months later.
The above photo, however, was taken on 3/10/77.

Patient: A.S.
Age: 5 years
Afflicted: 4 years

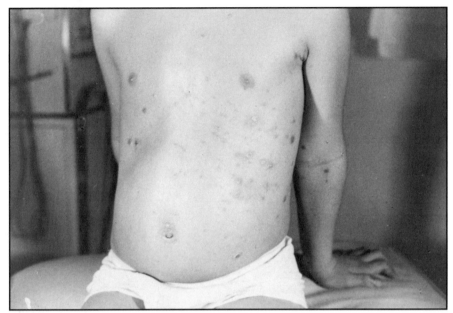

Fig. 2-7   Above photo was taken 1/13/77. Treatment was started 12/17/76.

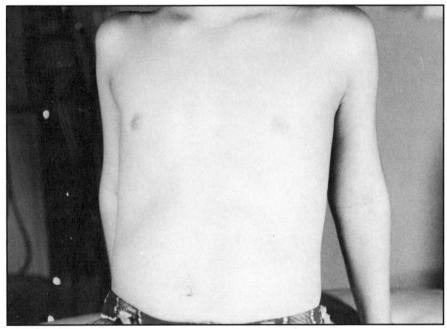

Fig. 2-8   Above photo taken 4/5/77—less than 4 months from start of treatment.

Patient: E.L.
Age: 8 1/2 years
Afflicted: 1 1/2 years

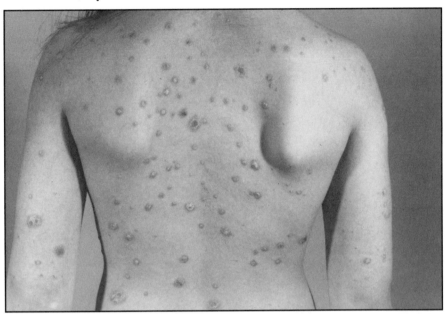

Fig. 2-9 Above photo taken 3/11/78—at start of treatment.

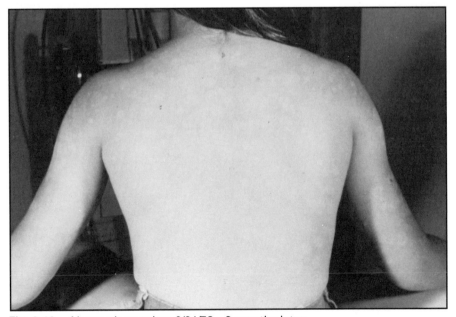

Fig. 2-10 Above photo taken 6/24/78—3 months later.

It soon become apparent to my patients and to me that we were truly on to something. When cases such as these continued to respond favorably, though in varying degrees, we could only conclude that we had been doing something right. The next step for me was to learn all I could about psoriasis from the orthodox as well as the Cayce point of view. Armed with the knowledge provided by both schools of thought, I devoted the next decade to treating patients with psoriasis, but only after medical procedures had been exhausted. The results of those years of research follow.

Chapter 3

About Psoriasis

It never fails to amaze me just how uninformed the average patient is about his skin, especially regarding his psoriatic condition. I can appreciate the fact that most individuals are mainly interested in ridding themselves of the disease without having to delve too deeply into the particular whys and wherefores. More than likely, I too would feel much the same way if I suffered from psoriasis. However, I submit that the patient's chances of achieving this goal are greatly enhanced if he or she is armed with even a smattering of knowledge as to what is actually happening to the skin. Even a minimum of insight and knowledge usually instills in a cooperative patient a desire to approach the prescribed regimen with discipline as well as enthusiasm. Having a physician tell a patient what to do is one thing, but making that patient actually understand the reasoning behind it is even more important. He will do what he is supposed to do and will know why he is doing it.

Before I continue to explain this new view and approach to healing psoriasis, I would like to review some known facts about the disease in order for my readers to acquire a more thorough understanding of what we are dealing with and the obstacles that must be overcome.

Psoriasis

Although the name of the disease is derived from the Greek, *Psora*, meaning "the itch", itching does not necessarily accompany psoriasis.

When it does, it can be devastating, but in general, I found that about half of the patients I have cared for were not particularly bothered by an itch.

Eczema, however, another common skin disease, is usually always accompanied by an itch. In a later chapter we will discuss the close link between eczema and psoriasis which is not ordinarily recognized. It may please the reader to know that once my patients were on the right course, the itch, whether from psoriasis, eczema or a combination of both, was the first symptom to disappear. This is the first sign that the process is working. It means that there is less surface activity. It then becomes a matter of time and persistence before the scaling stops, and the lesions eventually and gradually fade away.

What is Psoriasis?

Although not discernible to the human eye, the skin is always moving, changing, teaming with life, and constantly renewing itself. The functions of the skin are numerous, spectacular and miraculous. Without our being conscious of it, our skin protects us from harmful outside influences, prevents our losing vital internal elements, holds our body together, warns us of potentially harmful internal as well as external temperature changes, plays a major role in our immune system, and performs countless other functions. It also relays pleasurable sensations, beautifies our appearance when cared for, and in general equips us with the necessary protective barrier that enables us to live in this world.

That the skin constantly renews itself is an important factor to grasp, for here is where psoriasis enters the picture. Normally, the skin regenerates itself about once a month, roughly every twenty-eight days. In psoriasis, this process is speeded up; the skin attempts to renew itself every three or four days. One does not have to be a genius to realize that with such a deviation from the normal, something certainly is amiss.

Your Skin

Look upon your skin as having two basic layers. The deeper layer is called the derma or *DERMIS*, and carries all the blood vessels, nerves, glands, etc. where new skin cells are formed. The surface layer is called the *EPIDERMIS*, and is the harder, less delicate protective layer, covering the sensitive structures of the dermis.

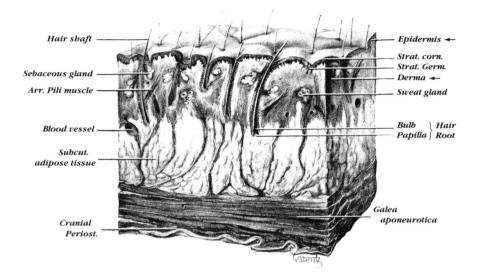

Hair shaft — Epidermis
Sebaceous gland — Strat. corn.
— Strat. Germ.
Arr. Pili muscle — Derma
— Sweat gland
Blood vessel — Bulb ⎱ Hair
Papilla ⎰ Root
Subcut.
adipose tissue
Galea
Cranial aponeurotica
Periost.

Fig. 3-1
Illustration showing a typical skin section

> From: *Gray's Anatomy* 26th Edition, Lea & Febiger Publishers, Philadelphia,
> PA., copyright 1954—Reprinted by permission. (30th Edition, Pub. in 1985,
> Edited by Carmine D. Clemente.)

Once the dermis forms new skin cells, they begin to migrate outward through various layers to form the cells of the epidermis. It takes about two weeks for these cells to move from the dermis to the epidermal layer. It then takes approximately another two weeks for the cells of the epidermis to die and gradually slough off. In the meantime, new cells have already replaced the old ones. In health, this process continues from birth to death, a marvel of bio-mechanical engineering.

When psoriasis is present, everything goes awry. The dermis tries to produce the new cells at an alarming rate. The surface area becomes red, inflamed, extremely sensitive, visibly raised and scaly. The specific area involved can rise to three times its thickness above the surface (Acanthosis).

A COMPARATIVE VIEW

Schematic comparison of (A) normal epidermis and (B) epidermis in psoriasis. Upward enlargement of dermal papillae permits up to three-fold increase of dermoepidermal area, which together with three-layered germinative cell layer accounts for nine-fold increase in germinative cell population. It is primarily this-increase that reduces the turnover time of the epidermis from a normal 28 days to 3 to 4 days.

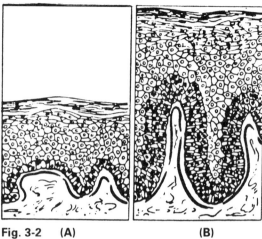

Fig. 3-2   (A)   **(B)**

From: *Dermatology In General Medicine*—Fitzpatrick et al, Pg. 221— Published by McGraw-Hill Book Company, ©1971, New York, N.Y. Reproduced by permission.

A psoriasis victim can form a scale so deep that peeling it off causes bleeding underneath. This is known as the "Auspitz" sign. The cells which are migrating to the surface under these conditions are obviously not normally effective in all of their functions because they have not had enough time to form completely; they are immature. Not only is the process unsightly, but it is unhealthy in that the normal functions of the skin are impaired, rendering the patient prone to internal as well as external environmental hazards.

In spite of all the research carried on since Robert Wilan of England recorded what seems to be the first accurate clinical description of psoriasis in 1808, the latest statement issued on the subject by the National Institutes of Health (NIH) says that "Scientists do not yet know what causes skin cells to reproduce so rapidly in psoriasis."[1]

To this I reply—let's take another look; this time from a different perspective—from the *inside out*, rather than from the outside in. From this new approach, we can more readily see why psoriasis lesions form on the surface of the body.

The Portals of Exit

Continuing to build on what we discussed in Chapter 1, we can now go one step further and learn that the toxins are emitted from the body via *the perspiratory system* (sweat glands).[2] Why toxins exit more readily in some areas rather than others is anybody's guess, for sweat glands are everywhere. There are about one hundred such glands in one square centimeter of skin surface, an area about the size of a little fingernail and approximately an eight of an inch thick.

There is a theory that lesions appear more frequently in areas of the body that are more subject to stress and strain, such as the elbows and knees. This view, however, does not hold true in all cases since many patients have lesions where there is no particular strain or trauma, for instance the abdomen or back.

The most common sites for lesions to form are the scalp, elbows, knees, small of the back, and lower legs. They can, however, appear literally anywhere, including under toenails and fingernails as well as on the sensitive inner linings of the mucous membranes. Why psoriasis shows itself here, there or everywhere is really immaterial when it comes to healing the disease.

Specific names have been given to the various types of psoriatic lesions. It must be remembered, however, that regardless of the varying degree of severity or the differences in appearance, *the disease is the same.* Many patients who followed the regimen presented in this book found that different kinds of lesions responded favorably even though they were treated basically the same way. Someone who has had the disease for twenty years cannot realistically expect to respond to treatment as fast as a person who has had it for only two months, although sometimes it is possible. Usually, the longer a person has had the condition, the greater the pollution of the system. Consequently, it will take *time* to clean out and replenish each cell of the body.

The Most Common Types of Psoriasis:

1. Common Vulgaris
2. Guttate
3. Flexural

4. Generalized/Erythrodermic

5. Pustular

6. Exfoliative

7. Psoriatic Arthritis

Common Vulgaris is sometimes referred to as "plaque-type" because it looks just as though a plaque had been pasted on the skin —as though it could simply be peeled off. The lesions are often quite noticeably raised, older lesions being darker in color and clearly circumscribed, with adjacent skin uninvolved. Many times, these separated plaques will come together, even during the healing process, and take on a generalized appearance. (See Color Photo Section —Case of J.R.)

Guttate lesions appear as little droplets on small or large areas of the body. Psoriasis often begins with this type in young people between the ages of eight and sixteen. A strep throat frequently precedes the first signs of the disease. Sometimes it will simply clear up by itself, or it can remain and advance to more severe stages.

Flexural psoriasis develops in the natural folds of the skin such as the armpit, breast folds, pubis, genital area, groin and buttock crease. The area affected appears highly inflamed, but without scales because of the body's natural lubrication. Since these sections are hardly ever exposed to the sun's rays, and medicated creams can prove most irritating, one can well imagine the joy of accomplishment when these lesions clear up by taking the internal approach described herein.

Generalized/Erythrodermic psoriasis is widespread, covering most of the body's surface. I have treated cases in which practically every square inch of the skin was affected. The body becomes red all over (erythro = "red") appearing almost like a boiled lobster. Scaling can be extensive, itching intolerable; and if arthritis accompanies the disease, the patient is faced with a double jeopardy. Can this form of psoriasis be healed naturally? It can be and has been, as is evident in the cases of A.M. and L.G. (See Color Photo Section).

Pustular psoriasis is a type in which pus forms on the lesions as it would on boils, indicating an infiltration of white blood cells. (See Color Photo Section —Case of J.C.) Although rare in itself, it can also become generalized, accompanied by fever and general debility. This is known as von Zumbusch's disease, after the physician who first described it. It is most common on the palms of the hands and soles of the feet. (See Color Photo Section—case of S.R.)

Exfoliative is the most devastating form of psoriasis. The entire skin is involved, and there is profound inflammation and scaling. It may result from an extension or advanced degree of acute guttate or other spreading eruptions. Exfoliative psoriasis usually ends with death in two or three years.[3]

Psoriatic Arthritis is a form of psoriasis accompanied by an erosive joint disease, sometimes severe, usually involving many joints, particularly the fingers. As the disease advances, demineralization of bone takes place which is readily discernible on x-ray examinations. Although it strongly resembles Rheumatoid Arthritis, blood tests reveal the absence of what is called the rheumatoid factor. Psoriatic Arthritis is therefore classified as a disease entity in itself. According to Dr. Ronald Marks, in his book *Psoriasis*, "Most surveys indicate that one person in twenty with psoriasis has some form of arthritis, and that about one person in twenty with arthritis has some form of psoriasis!"[4]

Age has little to do with this form of psoriasis. Some people develop it in their early teens. It is more prevalent in the twenties or thirties, but middle-aged people are also affected. Because of its importance, I have included a chapter, The Arthritic Connection, which deals exclusively with this form of the disease.

Most psoriatics know that the disease is noncontagious. This is not very comforting, however, in social or professional engagements when the condition is visible. Because of its physical appearance it is viewed by the average person as contagious and contact with the patient is usually avoided, especially in the case of strangers. This can lead to feelings of self-devaluation and embarrassment. Every effort is made to at least "look good"—and for many patients, that's good enough.

Of course, a patient may manifest one type of lesion that will eventually develop into another, or have different types that overlap each other. As previously mentioned, regardless of what form psoriasis takes, it is the same disease and the treatment is basically the same, with only minor variations. Strange as it may seem, I have seen some severe generalized cases clear up faster than others involving only one or two relatively minor spots. Whatever the extent or type, success was achieved only when the patients did not set a time limit, but simply followed the prescribed regimen and let nature take its course.

Statistical Data

Who is, or can be, afflicted with psoriasis? The answer to this question is plain and simple—anyone! Psoriasis is no respecter of age, color or sex. There are, however, certain groups in which it is more prevalent. The latest release by the NIH estimates the number of reported psoriatics in the USA alone to be approximately four to six million, with 150,000 new cases occurring each year. Worldwide, psoriasis afflicts about two percent of the population. In Sweden, however, for reasons yet to be determined, the figure is about three percent.[5]

The disease can manifest itself at any time, from infancy (although such cases are rare) to old age. The peak incidence, however, is between the ages of fifteen and thirty-five. Psoriasis appears in both males and females with equal frequency. Dark-skinned people are afflicted less frequently than fair or light-skinned individuals.

John O'Rourke's magazine article, "Vitamin A vs. Psoriasis," includes a list called "The Dermatologic Dozen" by Jerome Z. Litt, M.D., author of *Your Skin and How to Live In It*. Dr. Litt classifies psoriasis as the fourth most common skin disease exceeded only by acne, warts, and eczema, in that order.[6]

According to George Lewis, M.D., there is an associated family history in at least half of all psoriasis cases.[7]

Psoriasis is rare in North and South American Indians. It is common in East African natives and relatively rare in West Africans.[8] It is believed that the reason for the low incidence of psoriasis in American black people is due to their ancestral roots in West Africa. Japan is considered a country with a low incidence of the disease, but even there a significant number of citizens are afflicted.

I've often heard that European countries, especially Germany, showed a high incidence of psoriasis just prior to World War II. During the war the disease practically disappeared when food, especially red meats, were in short supply. After the war, as the economy recovered, and the food supply improved, there was also a concomitant resurgence of the disease. This in itself begins to tell us something.

In November 1989 I was asked to speak at the First International Conference on Holistic Health and Medicine in Bangalore, India, regarding the research I have conducted on psoriasis. It was the first time that I was able to get an idea of the incidence of psoriasis in the Far East. From the medical doctors who attended my lecture I learned that psoriasis, eczema and related skin diseases were widespread not only in India, but throughout Southeast Asia. They had a number of patients for me to examine as well as introduce to this new approach to healing the disease. Based on two percent of the 800 million population of India who are afflicted with the disease, we can safely assume that there are no less than 16 million psoriatics in India alone. This percentage is likely to be representative of all of Southeast Asia.

Assuming the statisticians are correct, two percent of the world's population (estimated at being five billion) would mean the number of people afflicted with psoriasis throughout the world approaches one hundred million! Of particular concern is the fact that psoriasis is on the increase, especially among the young.

Mechanisms that Trigger Psoriasis

Usually, a new victim of psoriasis first notices a small sore somewhere on the body, a sore that doesn't heal. It just seems to get worse and begin to spread. More sores then erupt in different areas. Some of the sores remain small or eventually disappear, but in most instances they get worse as time goes on, and the patient begins to seek relief.

There are occasions when the first signs of the disease appear after an injury or an abrasion of the skin. The damaged area does not heal properly and psoriatic lesions begin to develop along the site of the injury. This is known as the *Koebner Phenomenon*. Vigorous scrubbing, scratching, or picking at the area only makes it worse. Low humidity, systemically administered drugs, and severe emotional stress can also be triggering factors preceding the first outbreak of the disease.

There are many cases in which a pregnant woman with psoriasis seemingly improves during the gestation period. However, the disease usually returns after she delivers.

The fact is that the body is prone to being psoriatic long before the first signs of it appear. This is because internal pollution, the major causative factor of the disease, first affects the body on the *inside*.

Are Psoriatics Healthy?—A Personal Comment

Because psoriasis is rarely considered to be lifethreatening, it is often thought of by the scientific community as less important than other devastating diseases. In fact, one expert in the field of psoriasis research refers to most psoriatics as basically healthy people with a skin problem. I view this as a contradiction in terms. A psoriatic condition is the first sign that a patient is *not* in a healthy state.

One of my patients who had lesions on every square inch of his body said to me, "Doctor, I don't understand it. I am a healthy man—but look at me, I'm a mess!" And a mess he was—for twenty-five years. I am convinced that the word "healthy" is a total misnomer in a case like this. When discomfort, soreness, itching, cracking of the skin, etc. accompanies psoriasis, that patient indeed feels sick and unhealthy. I have had patients with massive lesions all over their bodies, but without discomfort, who looked upon their condition quite objectively and unemotionally. For some reason they were spared the painful irritation that often accompanies the disease.

In other words, when there are no perpetually distressing symptoms, it is not difficult for some people to live with this illness. When a patient is faced with irritating symptoms day in and day out, he is more inclined to seek relief by whatever means possible. But in either case, the patient is equally unhealthy and equally in need of treatment.

Therapies Available

The list of therapeutic measures developed over the years is long and varied. They encompass Topical (external), Systemic (internal) and Dual Therapy, such as Photochemotherapy (a combination of a drug with ultraviolet [UV] light). The results of the procedures also vary. With some patients they are often quite encouraging, while with others the response can be disastrous. Like anything else, some respond favorably, others do not. Practically every orthodox procedure involves some form of external application, usually in the form of salves, creams and lotions, but techniques ranging from tar baths to photochemotherapy to laser beams have been applied, again with varying degrees of success or failure. Ultrasound is experimentally used in some cases, as well as simple adhesive tape. Fluorinated steroids, steroid injections and Glucocorticosteroids (steroid compounds) are often used, but with careful monitoring, as the possible harmful side effects are well known. The side effects include thinning skin and redness and dilation of surface blood vessels.

The Goeckerman Regimen is one of the oldest and most effective therapies developed and was named after the American doctor who devised it. Discovered over 50 years ago, the Goeckerman Regimen consists of applying distilled tar, crude or refined, to the skin, leaving it on overnight in most cases and irradiating the skin the next morning with ultraviolet rays. Many times it clears the skin for long periods of time, but the "mess" involved is the greatest disadvantage to the patient. This method is used to this day as it has been proven to be moderately safe and effective.

PUVA refers to photochemotherapy. This type of therapy has been used experimentally for several years at The Massachusetts General Hospital. It is a combination of a drug, Psoralen, taken orally and followed in about two hours by carefully controlled exposure to Ultraviolet Light—Type A Therapy. Psoralen causes the skin to become more sensitive to the absorption of UV light. PUVA, although approved by the Federal Drug Administration (FDA) in May of 1982, has possible serious side effects such as the development of certain forms of skin cancer, cataract formation and an actual burn from the lights themselves. For these and other reasons, researchers use this form of therapy only in severe cases, and urge restraint in the long-term use of PUVA treatment.

Dialysis of the blood (Hemodialysis) is a treatment used to purify the blood of people with chronic kidney disease. It has been found, however, to help in cases of severe psoriasis, but again, the long-term effects are not yet known. It is used only as a last resort procedure.

Aromatic Retinoid is a drug chemically related to Vitamin A. It is a synthetic form of Vitamin A, remarkably effective in some severe cases. It should, however, be prescribed with care because, according to the National Institutes of Health, high doses can cause inflammation of the lips, hair loss and abnormal dryness of the eyes, skin and mouth.

Ultraviolet Light—Type A (UVA) by itself is not the best method of choice for clearing psoriasis. As mentioned earlier, when used extensively, it could have serious side effects. This type should only be applied in a dermatologist's office or a hospital setting.

Ultraviolet Light—Type B (UVB) is the most widely used light in the treatment of psoriasis, and has been used for over fifty years. A patient must build up a tolerance for it. Consequently, at first, small doses of about thirty seconds are applied and gradually increased. The effects are practically the same as normal sunlight. UVB light does not penetrate the skin as deeply as UVA.

Methatrexate (MTX), a cancer drug, is often used internally on the most severe cases. Liver biopsies, however, are routinely conducted on patients using MTX because after prolonged use the drug is known to have harmful effects on the internal (visceral) structures of the body, particularly the liver.

Etretinate (Tegison) is probably the latest drug (1986) available for treating psoriasis. It is a derivative of Vitamin A and has been experimented with widely in the United States and Europe. It is taken orally and can be used alone or in combination with other drugs and ultraviolet light treatment. It is used only in severe cases that have not responded to more conventional methods.

Activated Vitamin D Cream is the latest external application experimented with as of this writing (1990). According to Dr. Michael Holick, M.D., director of the Clinical Research Center at Boston University School of Medicine, a significant number of psoriasis cases responded quite favorably to Active Vitamin D and he hopes to gain FDA approval for its use, by prescription only, within a year. An oral form of Activated Vitamin D has already been approved, but it is not thought to be as effective as the topical form. Since this research is relatively new, to my knowledge, no statistics have been released as to its long-term effects.

The list of standard external salves, such as Anthralin (Dithranol), Psoragel, Estar, Salicylic Acid combined with coal tar or steroid cream, Diprosone, etc. is too long to mention. They all have their advantages and disadvantages, but whatever the methods used, they are palliative at best, masking the symptoms of an elusive disease that appears on the surface but originates elsewhere in the body.

Treatment at the Dead Sea—Lying in the deepest fault in the earth's crust on the border of Isreal and Jordan is the Mideast body of water known as the Dead Sea. Because of its extremely high salt content (nine times saltier than the oceans), nothing can live in it. Thus the name "Dead" Sea. For centuries, those who could afford to, traveled to the Dead Sea for cosmetic and health reasons claiming its waters cured psoriasis as well as arthritis and rheumatism.

Because the Dead Sea is 1,200 feet below sea level, there is a longer column of air through which solar radiation must travel. This filters out much of ultraviolet type B (UVB), leaving a higher amount of ultraviolet type A (UVA) light to which one is exposed, says Dr. Brian Diffey, principal physician, Dryburn Hospital, Durham, England. "However," he adds, "a person must sunbathe eight hours a day for three to four weeks at the Dead Sea to achieve clearance."

Also included as part of the therapeutic regimen is soaking in the Dead Sea, which may include various emollients and moisturizers that soften and peel heavy plaque-type psoriasis. In addition, it is believed that rest from the patient's stressful daily living and psychological group therapy aids in its effectiveness. Although medical authorities question its true value, tourists continue their pilgrimage to the Dead Sea for health reasons.

As this volume goes to press, The New England Journal of Medicine (Jan. 31, 1991—Vol. 324, No.5) released a paper by Ellis on the role *cyclosporine,* a new systemic treatment, has on severe plaque-type psoriasis. Cyclosporine was first noted to be effective in cases of psoriatic arthritis and psoriasis in 1979. There are, however, reservations as to its continued use since it has been suggested that long-term use of cyclosporine may lead to suppression of the natural immune system, systemic tumor (lymphoma) formations and because of the potential toxicity of the drug. The journal reports, "Thus, although cyclosporine is a highly effective agent for severe psoriasis, it should probably be used only as short-term therapy until more experience is reported."[9]

There Is Another Way

Surprisingly, most of my patients are quick to accept the idea that psoriasis is essentially an internal malfunction. Once this is explained, their reaction is, "It makes sense!" Rarely, if ever, have I met with resistance on a patient's part concerning this theory, especially after presenting them with tangible evidence of healing. For the first time since becoming afflicted they are given a possible explanation for their skin disorder which they can understand.

Armed with this new found knowledge, those patients who are open to it are ready to proceed—this time however, their attack on the problem will be launched from a different direction—a natural alternative.

REFERENCES

(Chapter 3—About Psoriasis)

1. *Fact Sheet on Psoriasis*, U.S. Department of Health, Education and Welfare, National Institutes of Health, DHEW Publication No. (NIH) 77-1104.
2. Edgar Cayce Reference # 3373-1, (Virginia Beach, VA, The Edgar Cayce Foundation, copyright 1971)
3. John Franklin, "Scaly Eruptions" in *French's Index of Differential Diagnosis*, ed. by Arthur H. Douthwaite, M.D., F.R.C.P. (Bristol, John Wright & Sons, Ltd., 1954, 7th Ed.) p. 732.
4. Ronald Marks, Dr., *Psoriasis*, (New York, NY, Arco Publishing, Inc. 1981) p. 32.
5. L. Hellgren, "Statistical, Clinical and Laboratory Investigation of 255 Psoriatics and Matched Healthy Controls," in *Psoriasis* (Stockholm, Acta Dermatovener, 44:191-207 1964.)
6. John O'Rourke, "Vitamin A vs. Psoriasis," *Let's Live* (April 1983) p. 24.
7. George M. Lewis, M.D., F.A.C.P., *Practical Dermatology*, (Philadelphia and London, copyright 1952, by W.B. Saunders Co.) p. 80.
8. A.R.H.B. Verhagen and J.W. Koten, *Psoriasis in Kenya*, (Chicago, Arch Derm 9639-41, 1967.)
9. Nicholas J. Lowe, M.D., "Systemic Treatment of Severe Psoriasis—The Role of Cyclosporine," *The New England Journal of Medicine*, Editorials, (Jan. 31, 1991,—Vol. 324, No. 5) pp. 333-334

Chapter 4

The Natural Alternative

The Regimen

The simple premise upon which this alternative approach to healing psoriasis is based is twofold:

    1. Clearing out the poisons that have accumulated in the body.

    2. Preventing further intake of toxic elements.

I say without reservation that once these two processes are set in motion, regeneration begins and new skin forms to replace the old.

Perhaps my readers will view this statement as rather bold, but I can attest to the fact that this is exactly what happens. The last chapter explained how new cells constantly form in the dermal layer of our skin and migrate to the outer layer to form the epidermis, which then sloughs off. This is an established scientific fact. Therefore, it is not inappropriate to say a "new" skin forms; it happens naturally, every month. The psoriatic's aim is that next time it will be new skin without the addition of toxic elements.

How long will it take for an individual to detoxify is impossible to determine. Each patient has his or her own built-in time clock. Keep in mind that it is the *direction* and not the *speed* that counts in this approach.

To achieve the two basic requirements stated above, the following measures are essential:

1. INTERNAL CLEANSING

2. A CLEANSING BUT NUTRITIOUS DIET

3. SPECIFIC HERB TEAS

4. ADJUSTMENTS OF THE SPINE

5. EXTERNAL APPLICATIONS

6. RIGHT THINKING—A *must* in the healing of any disease.

As we proceed, all of the above measures will be dealt with separately. Since each individual is different, certain measures will have more significance to some people than to others. Here is where the skill and sensitivity on the part of their physician or the patient's own personal perceptions come into play. In this way, the patient is able to determine his or her own strengths and weaknesses and proceed accordingly.

It will soon become obvious that this regimen not only makes you cognizant of your skin, but of your body as a whole. Many organs or systems of the body are dependent on one another. This is why something that benefits one system automatically benefits another and, conversely, something that breaks down one system can break down another. When on the right track, the body eventually reaches a state of equilibrium, becoming a full-fledged working unit of energy—the natural state of health.

Holistic Healing

Holism, or holistic healing, has become a household word. Man has evolved to the point of realizing that many things seen on the outside are actually formed or caused by things that are unseen. In considering holistic healing it is essential to recognize the human being as a unity of Spirit and Mind as well as Body. It is the proper balancing of these three aspects that constitutes the health and well-being of the individual.

Plato remarked in the *Phaedrus*, "For this is the great error of our day in the treatment of the human body, that the physicians separate the soul from the body." Only recently, many physicians have come to the same conclusion.

For instance, a skin disease may originate in an emotional upset, such as harbored resentments, and remain with a patient until the cause of the resentment is understood or eradicated. A headache has often been traced to a forgotten injury to the coccyx (tail bone) or to digestive disturbances caused by a poor diet. Improper absorption and assimilation of certain trace minerals can be the cause of mental illness, including some forms of schizophrenia. The Cayce material continually emphasizes this triune approach to health and encourages the balance of all three forces—Spirit, Mind and Body—as mandatory for our health and happiness, which is our birthright. This "Triune Principle", the balance of spirit, mind and body, is the basis of Holistic Healing and is the cornerstone upon which I conducted my research. In essence, it is properly setting in motion the forces of nature within the individual that will help the body heal itself.

The "1–2–3" Concept of the Disease

The results obtained over fifteen years of studying, observing and being actively engaged in the clinical management of psoriasis have led me to formulate what I call the "1-2-3" concept of the disease:

1. Psoriasis is the external manifestation of the body's attempt to eliminate internal toxins that have accumulated in the lymphatics and blood stream by "seeping" through thin intestinal walls.

2. It is characterized by inflamed patches (lesions) with silvery scales of skin that slough off in three to four days instead of the normal twenty-eight day period.

3. It is alleviated, controlled, or even possibly cured by taking the necessary steps to heal the intestinal walls and by opening up the normal channels of elimination as well as preventing further toxins from entering the system.

In the chapters that follow, I will help the reader further understand the basics of the disease from this new perspective. This will lead to viewing the healing of psoriasis as a *process* rather than a condition dependent upon a particular commodity; a process I call "The Natural Alternative."

NOTE TO MY READERS: THE READER SHOULD VIEW THE MATERIAL CONTAINED HEREIN AS A *REPORT* ON THE RESULTS OBTAINED WITH PATIENTS, BASED ON THE RESEARCH I CONDUCTED ON PSORIASIS. THIS INFORMATION SHOULD NOT BE REGARDED AS A GUIDE FOR SELF-DIAGNOSIS OR SELF-TREATMENT. CONSULTATION WITH YOUR PERSONAL PHYSICIAN PRIOR TO EMBARKING ON ANY THERAPEUTIC REGIMEN IS AN ABSOLUTE NECESSITY.

Chapter 5

Internal Cleansing

"Let's start at the very beginning—a very good place to start" are poignant lyrics from the ever delightful musical score of *The Sound of Music*.

What better place to begin our healing process than at the beginning? Common sense tells us to "clean house" before redecorating. In no uncertain terms, this is where the healing of psoriasis should commence.

There is nothing better than beginning fresh, unencumbered by pre-existing hindrances. In the case of psoriasis, the first condition to correct is the accumulated pollution that has infected the entire blood stream and, subsequently, all the organs and cells of the body. This is accomplished by opening up the normal channels of elimination: primarily, the bowels and kidneys, and secondarily, the skin and lungs.

Obviously, the most effective cleansing is obtained by clearing out the bowels and kidneys. This releases the "backup" pressure on the liver and gall ducts as well as the intestines, allowing free passage of their waste accumulations. In this way, the hepatic (liver) cells are free to perform one of their most important tasks; filtering out and purifying the blood and lymph.

Chronic constipation and *poor eliminative habits* are the major causes of colon impaction which in itself is one of the main reasons for the breakdown of the intestinal walls.[1]

In his classic medical textbook, *Symptoms of Visceral Disease*, Francis M. Pottenger, M.D. and world-renowned authority on neurology, clearly explains the effect a sluggish bowel has on the intestinal wall:

"When the contents of the intestinal tract are delayed in their movement through the intestine, they undergo certain changes which are more or less irritating and injurious to the intestinal wall. Stasis from this cause is usually accompanied by the absorption of toxins."[2]

This is why paying close attention to the colon and its proper functioning cannot be overemphasized.

THE COLON (Large Intestine):

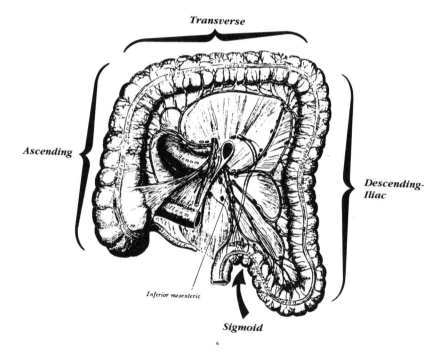

Fig. 5-1
The COLON is divided into four parts: the *Ascending, Transverse, Descending-Iliac* and *Sigmoid*.

Illustration from: *Gray's Anatomy*—26th Edition, Lea & Febiger Publishers, Philadelphia, PA., copyright 1954—Reprinted by permission. (30th Edition, Pub. in 1985, Edited by Carmine D. Clemente).

There are certain physical abnormalities that can cause a malfunction of the colon. Even if there is no pathological process such as a tumor formation or stricture, the colon, in some people, may be excessively lengthened beyond its normal five feet. This is called a "redundant" colon. Its positioning in the abdominal cavity may also be abnormal, causing an irregular twist or turn that slows down the normal passage of fecal matter.

The following illustration shows a few of the more common abnormal conditions that may occur in the colon. They are reproduced here through the courtesy of Dr. Bernard Jensen from his book *Tissue Cleansing Through Bowel Management*.

The following drawings illustrate some abnormal shapes of the bowel in comparison to a normal bowel.

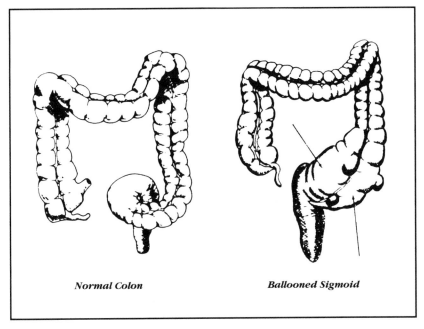

Normal Colon   *Ballooned Sigmoid*

Fig. 5-2A

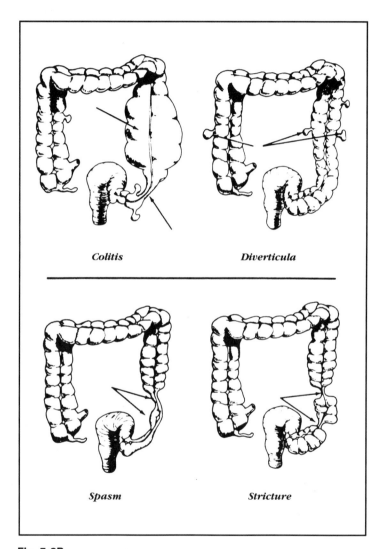

Fig. 5-2B

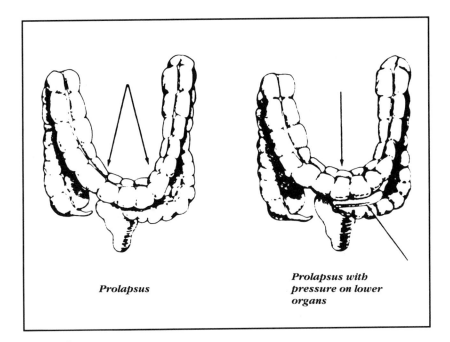

Prolapsus

Prolapsus with pressure on lower organs

Fig. 5-2C

Illustrations from: *Tissue Cleansing Through Bowel Management* by Dr. Bernard Jensen, D.C., Ph.D., and Sylvia Bell, copyright 1981, 6th ed., published by: Bernard Jensen, D.C., Route 1, Box 52, Escondido, CA 92025. Reproduced by permission.

In other words, there can be anatomical reasons for malfunction of the colon; it is not always a matter of poor diet or bad toilet habits. Whatever the reason for a malfunction, steps should be taken to correct it if at all possible. Fortunately, anatomical abnormalities are found in only a minority of cases. More often than not, the culprit in psoriasis is improper elimination due to poor eating habits, which in most cases can be corrected. Both require discipline on the part of the patient. With regard to eating, the patient should select easily digestible and more absorbable types of foods. Diet is dealt with quite thoroughly in Chapters 6 & Appendix A.

Bad toilet habits are more common than may be ordinarily suspected. It is quite amazing to discover what some people consider "normal." For instance, one patient, when asked about the frequency of his bowel movements, replied, "Oh, Doc!—I have no problem there; I go once every four or five days without fail!" Can you imagine the look of bewilderment on his face when I explained to him that having "no problem" meant eliminating once or preferably twice a day, if not more often? He had labored under a misconception for many years because a physician once told him that infrequent elimination was nothing to be concerned about, and that in his case, it was normal! Once his bowels were regulated to eliminating every day, his psoriasis, as well as other health problems that he faced, disappeared. Since then (eight years ago) he has never had a recurrence.

The reason for another patient of mine not eliminating more than once a week was, to quote her, "I didn't like going to the bathroom!" I eventually learned that this was a habit shared by all members of her family. She had actually been raised to believe that defecating was something "dirty" and should be done only when absolutely necessary.

Again, once she was convinced of the fallacy of such a ridiculous idea, she made it a point to alter her habits. In time, good results were evident in that her generalized psoriatic condition showed a gradual improvement. During one of the meetings of psoriasis patients I have held in my office, she remarked to other patients that she had not realized the beneficial effect regular bowel movements would have on her skin.

The principle to grasp here is that blockages or partial blockages of the colon, for whatever reason, are detrimental to the *general* well-being of the individual. The end result of such impairments may vary considerably, taking the form of one disease or another. The primary cause is often the same; only the name of the disease differs.[3]

Categorically speaking, rheumatoid arthritis, eczema, scleroderma, lupus erythematosus, psoriasis, and a number of other systemic diseases *may very well have the same basic cause.* The course of treatment is, therefore, essentially the same if the patient chooses the alternative route explained in this book. In these types of diseases, therapy should begin with INTERNAL CLEANSING, regardless of which disease it is. When this procedure is followed, the body can concentrate its efforts on rebuilding more quickly than if it had to destroy the "enemy"—i.e. the accumulated toxins—before starting reconstruction. It follows, then, that the more effective the internal cleansing, the quicker the disappearance of psoriasis.

The Kidneys

The Kidneys play as important a role in ridding the body of toxins as do the liver and bowel. They do so by filtering potentially dangerous impurities out of the blood and discarding them daily through the bladder in the form of urine. Each hour the blood filters through the kidneys twice. Vitamins, amino acids, glucose, hormones, etc. are returned to the bloodstream while excesses are eliminated in the urine. The end product of protein is *urea*. It is vital that the kidneys keep the level of urea in balance. If there is too little of it in the blood, it can indicate that the liver is not functioning properly; if too much, uremic poisoning of the blood can ensue, jeopardizing one's very life.

Many other functions are attached to the kidneys, such as helping the production of red blood cells, maintaining normal chemistry levels of the cells and playing a distinctive role in the acid/alkaline balance, a topic of utmost concern to the psoriatic.

Is it any wonder that the kidneys have been referred to often as the "master chemists" of the body? Keeping your kidneys cleansed and free of accumulated waste is accomplished principally by drinking an adequate amount of *pure* water daily. Six to eight glasses of water each day *in addition* to all other liquids is recommended. I often advocate that a patient keep a gallon of pure mountain spring water in the refrigerator at all times, and if desired, add the juice of a few *fresh* limes or lemons. This is not only a thirst-quenching drink, but also helps flush the kidneys and is alkaline reacting. In the next chapter we will discuss the significance of alkaline vs. acid reacting food and drink and how this relates to psoriasis.

[NOTE: In recent years, the condition of urinary incontinence (loss of bladder control) has become more recognized as a problem that affects ten million people in this country, mostly women. If they also happen to have psoriasis, they are faced with another problem since the recommendation of six to eight glasses of water daily would make life unbearable. Fortunately, there are medical procedures that have proven to be very effective, even curative. If such a problem exists, I highly recommend those patients have the condition of urinary incontinence corrected medically before proceeding with this regimen.]

THE KIDNEYS:

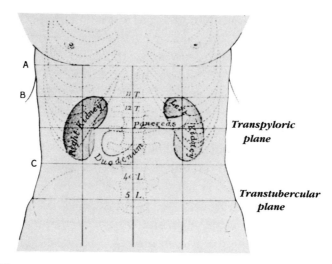

Fig. 5-3
Illustration showing position of the kidneys within the abdominal cavity

From: *Gray's Anatomy*—26th Edition, Lea & Febiger Publishers, Philadelphia, PA., copyright 1954—Reprinted by permission. (30th Edition, Pub. in 1985, Edited by Carmine D. Clemente.)

Dialysis, touched upon in my chapter "About Psoriasis", is a medical procedure used on kidney patients for the purpose of filtering out impurities in their blood when the kidneys no longer function properly. An interesting phenomenon has been observed in some kidney patients needing this form of therapy who also have psoriasis. It seems that they show a marked improvement in their skin when undergoing dialysis. Since the sole purpose of this medical procedure is to purify the blood, I think it is quite significant to note that the skin reacts in such a positive way when dialysis is administered. This interesting reaction was accidentally discovered years ago. Today, dialysis therapy is used on a limited basis, and only as a last resort, in extremely severe cases of psoriasis.

This obviously indicates that the kidneys play a significant role in keeping the skin free of blemishes when they function properly.

The Skin and Lungs

The skin and lungs are rarely recognized by the average person as an avenue of escape for toxins and impurities. They are, in fact, the secondary organs of elimination—second only to the bowel and kidneys. It is when we consider this function of the skin that we begin to recognize the reason for psoriasis lesions as well as the irritating, rash-like manifestation of eczema and other skin abnormalities.

The Skin: An illustration showing a typical skin section appears in Chapter 3. The sweat glands are discussed there in regard to how they function as portals of exit for accumulated toxins, thus fulfilling a major purpose of the skin. However, did you know that within that same one eighth inch square segment of skin (Chapter 3, Fig. 3-1) there are not only one hundred sweat glands but also twelve feet of nerves, hundreds of nerve endings, ten hair follicles, fifteen sebaceous glands and three feet of blood vessels?

In the eighteen square feet of skin that covers the body, there is a total of two million sweat glands. Each one is a tightly coiled little fifty-inch tube, buried deep in the dermis and rising out of it as a duct to the surface. In total, there are six miles of these ducts. These sweat glands function almost continually, extracting water, salt and *waste* from the blood. Is it any wonder that the skin is the largest organ in the body?

The Lungs: Most people fail to appreciate the connection there is between the lungs and the removal of internal toxins. The specific function of the lungs is to take air from the external environment, oxygenate the blood to be distributed throughout every body cell, and remove gaseous poisons, particularly carbon dioxide, from the body. Deep breathing exercises, such as those taught in yoga, have proven how pure air, properly inhaled, retained for a short time, and exhaled slowly, greatly improves the physical and mental health of an individual.

In a normal state of health, one is hardly cognizant of the lungs. In fact, it has been said that when you are aware of your lungs, you are already in trouble!

The lungs normally pump in and out about seventeen times a minute. Walking requires more oxygen, so the pumping increases to approximately twenty-four breaths per minute. Running doubles that amount to about fifty breaths. When exercise is conducted in the open air, the blood's used gases are expelled and replaced by oxygen more freely; hence exposing the lungs to impurities such as chemical fumes and automotive exhaust should be avoided if at all possible. The psoriatic should be aware of these facts and act accordingly, for by purifying the lung fields a major step is taken to rid the body of psoriasis.

THE LUNGS:

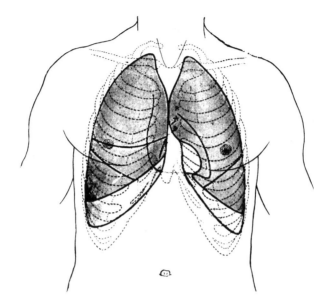

Fig 5-4
Illustration showing position of lungs in thorax

From: *Gray's Anatomy*—26th Edition, Lea & Febiger Publishers, Philadelphia, PA., copyright 1954—Reprinted by permission. (30th Edition, Pub. in 1985, Edited by Carmine D. Clemente.)

Take care of your lungs, nurture them by supplying them with the fresh air they need in order to function properly. They will, in turn, take care of every cell, organ and muscle in your body, supplying you with oxygen for every activity from sleeping to running to thinking. Guard these sentinels of vital energy well, for your lungs truly provide you with the breath of life.

The Liver

The liver is so remarkable an organ that some cultures regard it as the site of life. One cannot begin to understand how the body filters out toxic elements without an appreciation of the incredible task carried out by the liver.

THE LIVER:

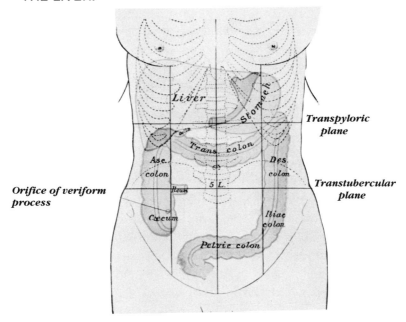

Fig. 5-5
Illustration showing position of the liver in relation to other structures of the abdominal visera

From: *Gray's Anatomy*—26th Edition, Lea & Febiger Publishers, Philadelphia, PA., copyright 1954—Reprinted by permission. (30th Edition, Pub. in 1985, Edited by Carmine D. Clemente.)

When the liver is not functioning properly, not only do toxins build up in the body, but as a consequence, changes in mood, behavior and general health can occur. It has been determined that the liver is responsible for over 500 separate activities. Of these various functions, the one we are most concerned with is the *breakdown and excretion of poisonous materials*. The liver is one of the major filtering glands of the body. Its many functions, believe it or not, are primarily carried out by a single, remarkable structural unit called the hepatic cell. There are approximately 300 billion of these unique cells in one liver which, among other things, filters two and one half pints of blood per minute when the body is at rest. In one year, it amounts to filtering out enough blood to fill twenty-three milk trucks! The liver has remarkable regenerative powers as well. If ninety percent of the liver was removed, the remaining piece could still function; in fact, it might even grow back to full size.

As miraculous as the liver is in its makeup and functions, it can nevertheless reach a breaking point by constant abuse and overtaxation. Barring direct injury to the liver and/or pathological processes, the most common reason for liver depletion is improper diet or liquid intake. When the liver becomes too seriously overtaxed with the resulting toxins, a breakdown of hepatic cells occurs, thereby opening the door to malfunction, infection and congestion.

Fortunately, the liver, as stated earlier, has incredible regenerative powers when given the right fuel to work with. It behooves us, therefore to do all in our power to keep this vital organ pliable and free of accumulated toxins. One of the most understandable ways of accomplishing this, obviously, is to prevent destructive food items from entering the system at all, hence the importance of proper nutrition. Patients should do well by eating or drinking items that have a known internal cleansing effect, such as those recommended in Chapter 6 and Appendix A which deal with Diet and Nutrition.

In order to regenerate the liver by external means, one of the most effective measures is to gently but thoroughly massage the entire liver area with an olive oil/ peanut oil mixture. [See illustration of liver—Fig. 5-5]

Another effective procedure I suggest to some patients is the application of warm Castor Oil packs directly over the liver. The simplest way this is accomplished is by saturating the liver area with Castor Oil and placing a warm, damp, soft cloth (preferably white flannel, four layers in thickness) over this area, and then covering the area with a piece of plastic wrap. A heating pad, set at medium, is then placed over the entire pack for approximately one to two hours. I have found to my satisfaction that massaging the liver or applying hot Castor Oil packs to it are among the healthiest measures that can be taken to help this organ perform its function of purifying the blood.

The Liver/Skin—Kidney/Lung Correlation

There have been many theories put forward as to the effect internal pollution has on the body, but when it comes to skin and lung disorders, none can compare with the work of Henry G. Bieler, M.D., in his excellent book, *Food Is Your Best Medicine*. I suggest that my readers carefully read the following passage from this book, for it provides the basic information needed for an understanding of the Liver/Skin—Kidney/Lung connection.

"The liver and the kidneys are important eliminative organs. For the liver, the natural avenue of elimination, of course, is through the bowel; for the kidneys, through the bladder and urethra.

However, when the liver is congested and cannot perform its eliminative function, waste matter (toxins) is thrown into the bloodstream. Similarly, when the kidneys are inflamed, toxins are also dammed up in the blood. Toxic blood must discharge its toxins or the person dies, so nature uses vicarious avenues of elimination or substitutes. The lungs, therefore, will take over the task of eliminating some of the wastes that should have gone through the kidneys, or *the skin will take over for the liver*. It stands to reason that the lungs do not make very good kidneys. From the irritation caused by the elimination of poison through this "vicarious" channel, we can get bronchitis, pneumonia or tuberculosis, as is determined by the particular CHEMISTRY of the poison being eliminated. Thus, we can say that the lungs are acting VICARIOUSLY for the kidneys or are being called into play, under duress, as substitute kidneys. In the same way, if the bile poisons in the blood come out through the skin, we get the various irritations of the skin, resulting in the many skin diseases, or through the mucous membranes (inside skin) as the various catarrhs, or through the skin as boils, carbuncles, acne, etc. *Thus, the skin is substituting for the liver, or a vicarious elimination is occurring through the skin.*"[4] [Emphasis added.]

From the quotation above, I am sure you can appreciate the fact that one part of the body cannot be separated from another. They are all interconnected. Polluting one area spills over to pollute another; conversely, by purifying one area, you purify another. The proper goal for psoriatics is to purify the *entire* system. When this is accomplished, no matter how long it takes, the inner condition of cleansed body cells will be reflected in the outer appearance of the body's surface—a healthy looking skin.

EFFECTIVE CLEANSING MEASURES

Since the primary organs of elimination are the bowels and kidneys, it is important to concentrate on their proper functioning and the measures that will help to purify them. The effectiveness of the diet, teas, adjustments, oils, etc., will increase a hundredfold if the body is kept internally cleansed. By doing so, one begins fresh, renewing the body even down to the cellular level. In my opinion, the initial cleansing is the turning point in psoriasis—*the point when the disease process begins to reverse itself.* As soon as body pollutants are no longer assimilated, and a cleansing diet is followed, detoxification will begin to take place.

As purification takes hold, more and more toxins exit every cell in the body. When this stage is reached, nutritious food elements are assimilated properly and the rebuilding begins on a cellular level. It is only a matter of time before complete renewal occurs, provided of course, the condition has not reached the point of no return.

The toxins produced by the body "sludge" are removed primarily by ingesting laxative foods and drinks and by cleansing the large intestine (colon). In addition, perspiration induced by taking a steam bath, coupled with deep breathing exercises, is also beneficial in removing toxic elements from the skin itself and also from the lung fields. An adequate amount of cleansing fluids taken daily will help to insure kidney purification. These are the processes by which the body rids itself of accumulated toxins. For greater effectiveness, a colonic irrigation or home enema should be *preceded* by a cleansing diet, several of which will be discussed later in this chapter.

The High Colonic Irrigation

With regard to the bowel (colon), there is, in my estimation, no more effective cleansing measure devised by modern man than the *high colonic irrigation* or high enema. It is best described as a gentle, effective method of hydrotherapy used to cleanse the large intestine. The high colonic cleans out the sigmoid, descending, transverse, and ascending colon, which, in total, measures approximately five feet in most adult individuals. [See Fig. 5-1] Fecal matter and waste can accumulate over a period of years around the inner lining of the colon. Since numerous lymphatics are directly attached to the outer walls of the colon, toxic matter constantly feeds the lymphatic attachments and invades the lymphatic chain. A properly administered high colonic irrigation is capable of flushing out impacted waste matter that has adhered to the inner walls of the large intestine. Once this is accomplished, the impurities will have been flushed out; consequently, the "seepage" of toxins will no longer occur.

The ultimate benefit, as I see it, is that it relieves the tendency toward chronic constipation, thereby aiding in preventing intestinal stasis (an undue delay in the passage of fecal matter along the intestines), which was referred to earlier in a quotation from the medical researcher, Francis M. Pottenger, M.D.

A *properly administered* high colonic can often mean the difference between success and failure for the psoriatic. I stress "properly administered" because a good technician, experienced in high colonic therapy, is not easy to find, and the sanitary conditions of the unit itself are as important as the technique applied. It is of the utmost importance that strict sanitary conditions prevail wherever colonics are administered. Even though the bowel may not be considered a sterile area, it should be cleansed with sterile equipment in order to avoid contamination. If the therapist who administers the colonic, usually an R.N., is reputable and maintains his or her equipment according to strict professional requirements, there should be no problem. If a patient feels apprehensive about either the condition or appearance of the unit or qualifications of the technician, they are advised to excuse themselves under the guise that they will have to give it more thought. I advise them not to return if there is any question about the professionalism of the technician or sanitary conditions of the unit.

In recent years, disposable nozzles and hoses have become available. They are used on a patient only once and then discarded. It goes without saying that the chances of infection are greatly reduced, and in fact are practically nonexistent when disposables are used.

After recommending high colonics for over thirty years, I conclude that a truly competent high-colonic therapist is as valuable in the restoration of health as a highly skilled surgeon. Although the procedure is not as admired, and the techniques not as involved, the *value* of a colonic can at times be immeasurable. In some cases it may even help to avoid surgical intervention. In severe or stubborn psoriatic/eczema conditions, I do not hesitate to recommend this form of hydrotherapy.

One of my patients who had been on the regimen for two months without any appreciable results, thus failing to respond as quickly as I had expected, took heed of my prodding and had two colonic irrigations in one week. Results were almost immediate. She began to clear up quickly, and within two more months, her skin was free of all lesions. It has remained so ever since. She remarked to me that the turning point was when she had these two colonic irrigations. It was from that moment that she "knew" she was going to be well. (See case of M.F., Color Photo Section.)

The way in which opponents of the colonic irrigation reach out to extremes in order to prove their point never fails to amaze me. They talk of the *possibility* of bowel rupture, the *possibility* of bowel infection, the *possibility* of destroying the bacterial flora necessary for normal bowel function. Their biggest argument seems to be that the patient may become dependent on colonics from overuse.

To say that these possibilities do not or cannot exist is just as ridiculous. Of course they exist—but so do surgical mishaps occur, as do dangerous side effects from drugs, despite taking all necessary precautions. Statistically, there is far less chance of any harm befalling a patient from a colonic than from drugs or surgical procedures. The admitted "potential" dangers of MTX (Methotrexate) as well as PUVA (Photochemotherapy) are well-known and well-documented, yet both are widely used in leading psoriatic centers as well as in private practices.

My patients have only a few colonics over a seven or eight-week period. Then they are followed-up by a colonic once every few months until the psoriatic condition clears. As a maintenance measure, one more after another six months is administered if need be. Nevertheless, a colonic should only be administered under the approval of a patient's personal physician.

High colonics are not advised for children or teenagers under 16. In such cases I recommend gently applied home enemas simply using warm water with a "ball" syringe.

Home Enemas

If for any reason a patient cannot have a high colonic, I advise a home enema. The difference between a high colonic and a home enema is that an enema usually cleans only the descending and sigmoid segments of the colon (about ten to twelve inches), while the high colonic cleans out the transverse and ascending colon as well (a total of about five feet in most individuals) as noted earlier.

Another obvious difference is that a professional colonic, in most cases, must be performed by an operator at a specific time and at a designated facility, whereas a home enema may be applied in the privacy of one's own home when it is convenient. Lastly, there is the expense to be considered, especially if several are required. Colonics can cost anywhere from $50 to $75 each, depending upon your location. A home enema, unless administered by a professional, is nominal in cost.

A Patient's Technique for a Home Enema

I include here a technique developed by one of my former psoriasis patients who suffered from the disease for over twenty years. As a result of applying this method faithfully, her skin condition improved dramatically.

She would lie on her back on the bathroom floor or in the bathtub and administer a home enema and retain the water in her colon for as long as possible before evacuating. While in this position, she would do gentle exercises, i.e. knee to chest, elbows to knees, upside-down bicycle, etc., and then lie back with her knees up and massage the area of the colon, from side to side. This is a most effective way to stimulate the peristaltic action of the colon as well as break away any fecal accumulations that may exist on the walls of the colon.

The lady warns, "Be ready to abandon ship at a moment's notice!" but advises that "after a few practice sessions, anyone can do it easily." She administered the enema on an average of twice a week.

After following this procedure for four months, as well as the additional measures in the regimen, she found the massive psoriatic areas on her back greatly improved, with no remaining scars. After this period of time, enemas were no longer required. Photographs taken two years later showed further improvement. (See Color Photographic Section—Case of L.G.)

Preliminary Diet to the Colonic or Home Enema

In order to insure the maximum cleansing of toxins from the system, the colonic or enema should be *preceded* by following the *Three-Day Apple Diet*. From the standpoint of economy, convenience, and practicality, I have opted to modify the original instructions suggested in the Cayce material for my patients as set forth below.

Modified Three-Day Apple Diet

DAY ONE

First thing in the morning: drink a glass of warm water to which the juice of one fresh lemon has been added.

An hour later, begin the following: Throughout the day, drink plenty of water and eat as many apples (Red Delicious or Yellow Delicious) as desired. Most of my patients eat approximately six to eight apples on the first day of this diet.

Late in the afternoon or in the evening: if at all possible, a high colonic is recommended; if not, a thorough home enema is advised. The purpose of having an enema at this time is to clear out the toxins that have already begun to accumulate in the lower intestinal tract. *In the evening*, they drink one tablespoon of pure olive oil, either plain or mixed in hot water or apple juice.

NOTE: If a full tablespoon of olive oil upsets their stomach, I recommend that the amount be reduced to one teaspoon. Even this amount may be intolerable if one suffers from either a gallbladder or liver condition. Whatever the case, they omit the olive oil if adverse reactions occur.

DAY TWO

They repeat all instructions given for Day One, except that a home enema is recommended instead of a high colonic.

DAY THREE

Again, they repeat all instructions given for Day One. It is most important that a high colonic or enema be given at the end of Day Three.

At the completion of this three-day cycle, they eat a pint of *plain* yogurt which will help to replace the normal bacterial flora of the intestinal tract. *An hour later*, if hunger persists, they may commence following the dietary suggestions outlined in Chapter 6 and Appendix A which allow a greater variety of foods.

Apples—Not for Everyone

Without question, some people cannot tolerate apples, raw or cooked, no matter how they are prepared. Apples can cause intestinal discomfort or severe allergic reactions. If this is the case, the Apple Diet should not even be attempted. There are those, however, who can tolerate apples to a certain degree, but not for three days. Under these circumstances, I recommend going on the diet for *one full day* instead of three days, and in the evening taking one tablespoon of olive oil. On the next day, I recommend either a home enema or a high colonic.

If, during this cleansing period, a patient experiences weakness, dizziness, or any other adverse reactions, I take him off the Apple Diet and replace it with the more liberal cleansing diet discussed in Chapter 6 and Appendix A. Such weakness or dizziness may be the result of a drop in blood sugar. These reactions are often relieved immediately by drinking a glass of orange juice, taking a tablespoon of pure honey, or eating a small portion of yogurt.

At the end of either the One-Day or the Three-Day Diet, the patient then proceeds by following the dietary measures set forth in Chapter 6 and Appendix A.

Alternatives to the Apple Diet

For those patients who *know* they cannot tolerate apples and are allergic to them, there are alternatives—*The Grape Diet*, *The Citrus Diet*, and *The Fresh Fruit Diet*. The steps in these diets are almost identical to those in The Apple Diet.

The Grape Diet

On this diet, they may eat as many grapes as desired for *three days* and should drink at least six to eight glasses of pure water *daily*. Almost any type of grape may be eaten, but I recommend the black Concord variety.

Late in the afternoon or evening on the *first* and *second* days of this diet, a thorough home enema is advised. In addition, *each evening*, one tablespoon of pure olive oil should be taken, either plain or mixed in hot water, grape juice, or any other fruit juice. On the *third* day, one should have a professionally administered high colonic late in the afternoon or evening, if possible. Again, a thorough home enema may be substituted. This is to be followed by consuming a pint of plain yogurt. One hour later, the patient may proceed with the dietary suggestions outlined in Chapter 6 and Appendix A.

The Citrus Diet

The Citrus Diet consists primarily of tropical and subtropical fruits. The most common of these are oranges, grapefruit, lemons, limes, tangerines, kumquats, mandarin, tangelo and pomelo. This diet should be followed for *five days instead of three*. One may eat an unlimited amount of these specific fruits, in addition to drinking six to eight glasses of pure water daily.

The ideal procedure would be to have a high colonic administered late in the afternoon or evening of the *first and fifth day*, and on the *third day* a home enema. If high colonics are not available, I suggest having home enemas on the *first, third and fifth day*. Each evening, one tablespoon of pure olive oil should be taken either plain, mixed with hot water, or mixed with any other citrus fruit juice.

At the end of the five-day cycle, a pint of plain yogurt should be consumed, and after one further hour, the patient should commence the dietary measures outlined in Chapter 6 and Appendix A.

NOTE: As in the case of apples, some people are hypersensitive to citrus. If such is the case they are to avoid the citrus diet.

The Fresh Fruit Diet

The fresh fruit diet is exactly what the name implies. All fruits may be eaten in any quantity on a daily basis, in addition to all the pure water that one can drink. This diet is maintained for a period of either three or five days.

The advantage of choosing this diet as opposed to the others is that it is more filling and satisfying, offers greater variety, and that the fresh fruits may be eaten either raw or cooked. The only stipulation as to the choice of fruits, according to the Cayce material, is that all varieties of melons, raw apples and bananas must be eaten separately rather than mixed with other fruits. Strawberries should not be eaten if there is an underlying arthritic condition.

If a patient chooses the three-day fruit diet, a home enema should be applied late in the afternoon or in the evening of the *first* and *second* day and a high colonic applied on the *third*. If it is not possible to get a colonic, another home enema may be substituted.

If a patient follows the five-day diet, a high colonic or home enema should be administered on the *first* and *fifth* day. A pint of yogurt is to be consumed after the *last* colonic or enema; one hour later, the patient is permitted to begin a more varied and satisfying diet with the foods designated in Chapter 6 and Appendix A. During this three or five-day period, a tablespoon of pure olive oil is taken each evening.

These diets not only rid the body of an enormous amount of toxins, but a patient can also expect a weight loss of approximately five to six pounds or more.

NOTE: If either dizziness or weakness occurs during this cleansing period, or if a patient continues to have hunger pangs, I advise adding either a large green leafy salad or a scoop of lowfat cottage cheese, lowfat yogurt, or sugarless jello to the diet. These additional foods help to provide more bulk.

If there is any question as to whether or not a patient can follow any of these cleansing diets, I insist they consult with their medical doctor before commencing. Some patients may not be able to follow these diets safely if they have, in addition to psoriasis, an underlying diabetic, hypoglycemic, candida or diverticulitis condition.

The Importance of Water

When one realizes that the body is primarily made up of water, it is not hard to fully recognize how vital this element is to all of the body's chemical processes. This is a biological fact from birth to death. In the embryo, water constitutes ninety percent of the body's weight. In the adult, water makes up seventy-three percent, discounting fat. As one gets older, the percentage diminishes even more. In general, it is safe to say that your physical body is always two thirds to three quarters water.

Without this universal medium in which all living biological transactions occur, life is not possible. Among other things, it is the most important cleansing element of the body: the tissues are bathed, the intestines are purified, the body temperature is regulated, and the body humors are maintained. Other functions, too numerous to mention, are dependent upon body water. Obviously, water intake is of the utmost importance in internal cleansing. Our water intake is derived primarily from food, sec ondarily from beverages, and lastly from the oxidation processes, such as fat burning, which produces a lesser amount of water, but is nonetheless a major source.

To repeat: *The recommended daily intake of water is six to eight glasses*, in addition to all other liquids consumed. Water should be drunk *before* and *after* meals, which will not only insure proper digestion, but will also help flush the kidneys, thereby draining accumulations of uric acid.

Needless to say, the *purer* the water the better. Because of all the various chemical additives in city water today, plus the continued pollution of our natural water sources, I recommend a home water filtering system or any mountain spring water that is considered to be pure.

Natural Cathartics (Laxatives)

A cathartic is a purgative used to produce an evacuation of the bowel. Some are medicinal in their makeup, while others are natural. It is the latter type that I deal with and, when necessary, strongly advise my patients to use. While the colonic or enema cleans out the large intestine or colon, the natural cathartic cleans out the upper intestinal tract as well. Combined, these two methods are the most effective procedures to cleanse the entire alimentary canal, from stomach to bowel.

Nature's best cathartics are raw fruits and vegetables. Stewed fruits are also quite effective and should be eaten as often as possible. The most beneficial fruits for stewing are figs, apples, raisins, apricots, pears, peaches and prunes. They may be mixed together if desired and are to be eaten until a complete evacuation takes place. Thereafter, making stewed fruits part of one's daily diet will help to keep the system cleansed, and at the same time supply the body with natural sugars.

In the case of fruits with a seedy nature, i.e. figs, raisins, etc., the intestinal movements are mechanically stimulated by the action of the indigestible portion of the fruit residue (seeds). These seeds stimulate local reflexes in the nerves of the intestinal walls. The skins from fresh fruit and the cellulose from raw vegetables, whole wheat and bran all serve as intestinal stimulants by increasing bulk, and consequently the degree of stretch of the walls of the bowel.

Foods rich in Vitamin B are especially advised, not only because of the nutritional value they provide, but because of the little-known fact that

Vitamin B aids in cleansing the bowel. From *The Living Body*, by Best and Taylor, we learn:

> "Vitamin B, and other factors of the B Complex, tend to increase the tone of the intestinal musculature, and thus favor natural movements of evacuation."[5]

According to modern nutritionists, foods rich in Vitamin B and B Complex include wheat germ, brewer's yeast, whole raw barley, soybean flour, whole wheat flour, buckwheat, raw peas, egg yolks, rye bread, almonds, fish, poultry, honey, turnips, beets, dandelions, leafy green vegetables, and broccoli.

Effective Combinations

Senokot, a natural vegetable laxative derived from the Senna Leaf, in granular form, is a natural, non habit-forming cathartic. A teaspoon of Senokot mixed in a glass of *warm* prune juice is an exceptionally effective laxative. I advise some of my patients to drink this combination at least once a day until they have a complete evacuation. Prune juice is not recommended, however, for those who are diabetic. If this is the case, Senokot should be mixed in a glass of *warm* water.

Fletcher's Castoria, when combined with the syrup made from California figs, is another excellent eliminant. One teaspoon of Castoria should be removed from a six-ounce bottle and replaced with one teaspoon of syrup of figs. From a twelve ounce bottle, two teaspoons should be removed and replaced with two teaspoons of the syrup. Before being taken, the bottle is well shaken. My patients then take a half-teaspoon of this mixture every half hour until they have a complete evacuation.

Alternating Castoria and syrup of figs by taking them separately is also an effective method. In other words, a patient takes a half teaspoon of Castoria, then one half to one hour later half-teaspoon of syrup of figs. This cycle should be continued until a complete evacuation occurs.

[NOTE: Syrup of figs was prepared by soaking 5 or 6 California Figs in a pot of cold water for a few hours. The water completely covered the figs by 4 or 5 inches. The water was brought to a boil, then reduced to simmer the figs, with the cover on, for approximately 50 minutes. If too much evaporation took place after 15 minutes, more water was added. The figs

were eaten as stewed and the liquid (syrup) placed in a jar and refrigerated after cooling.]

Orange Juice Sandwich: For centuries, Castor Oil has been a well-
known, effective purger of toxins from the body. For those who find it difficult to take by itself, the way to make it not only effective but also
palatable is to combine it with orange juice. Two ounces of orange juice
is poured into a six-ounce glass, then the glass is tilted and one ounce of
Castor Oil is slowly added to the orange juice. This is then followed by
another two ounces of orange juice. The Castor Oil will remain suspended
between the two layers of orange juice, thus making an "orange juice
sandwich." Taking Castor Oil in this manner makes it easier to swallow.
Apple juice may be substituted for orange juice and olive oil or cod liver
oil may take the place of Castor Oil.

Zilatone, *Innerclean* and *Psyllium Husks* are additional eliminants
that are recommended. These products are sometimes available in health
food stores, and can be purchased through the Cayce Product Suppliers,
listed in Appendix C.

Eno Salts, a fruit-based product, is another natural laxative recommended, as are *Upjohn's Citrocarbonates* and *Milk of Magnesia*, which
are alkaline in nature.

There are many more safe, non-habit-forming eliminants on the market today. For the best results, it is advisable to alternate them by using a
vegetable-based eliminant on one day and a fruit-based eliminant on
another day.

Olive Oil

Olive oil, taken by itself, is a very practical and effective cathartic. I
advise my patients to take a half-teaspoon of olive oil approximately three
or four times a day until it produces a good bowel movement. If one has a
gallbladder condition, smaller doses are suggested.

Olive oil, taken internally, has recently been recognized by the scientific community as being effective in preventing cholesterol buildup on the
arterial walls. This oil has also been credited with supplying nutrients to
the digestive tract, aiding in elimination, and acting as an intestinal food.

As a gentle enema, olive oil is also recommended for a thorough
cleansing of the colon. In order to relax the colon, applying a home

enema using a half-pint of pure olive oil with no other additives is often effective. After a complete evacuation occurs, a follow-up enema using *warm* water is suggested. As a final rinse, one tablespoon of Glyco-Thymoline (an alkaline cleansing mouthwash) should be added to a quart and a half of *body temperature* water. This final cleansing measure will prevent a generalized "weakening" state. I recommend this procedure be carried out by my patients once or twice a week, especially in either chronic cases of constipation or stubborn psoriatic conditions.

The Tri-Salts

This mixture has been advised in the Cayce readings as another effective cleansing agent for psoriasis sufferers. It is made up of the following:

Sulphur ....1 Tablespoon
Cream of Tartar............1 Tablespoon
Rochelle Salts...............1 Tablespoon

This product is sold through the Cayce supplier outlets in Virginia Beach, VA. under the trade name "Purilax" from Home Health Products, Inc., and as "Sulflax" from the Heritage Store, Inc. [See Appendix C]. Patients who decide to use it are advised to take one teaspoon every morning as directed on the label. Although Purilax and Sulflax are non-prescription items, they should be administered under the direction of an osteopath or medical doctor.

High Fiber Foods

The importance of high-fiber foods in today's diet cannot be overemphasized. These foods are highly advisable, for they help to stimulate peristaltic action throughout the intestinal tract and cleanse the colon by virtue of their coarse action on the walls.

The past decade has brought about new awareness of the value of high-fiber foods in the prevention of cancer of the colon. The *New England Journal of Medicine* published a report stating that researchers at the University of Modena in Italy believe that high-fiber foods possibly prevent cancer of the colon, as well as heart disease, by lowering blood levels of cholesterol. One reason for this, the researchers believe, is that high-fiber diets speed up the movement of food through the small intestines, thereby preventing certain disease processes from "taking hold." The Associated Press released an article in June 1982 reporting findings by a panel of scientists, based on a two-year study, for the National Academy of Sciences, indicating that a diet high in fiber supplied by wholegrain cereals, fruits and vegetables may inhibit certain cancers.

Although these scientists claim that their findings are inconclusive, the fact remains that fiber-rich foods have a cleansing effect throughout the colon because of their inability to be digested. Fibrous-type foods (roughage) speed up the process of waste elimination, and the destructive, possibly even cancerous, elements do not have time to gain a foothold in the large intestine before they are "scraped" off the walls of the colon and passed out of the body. These conclusions parallel those of the researchers from the University of Modena.

The most common high-fiber foods are whole or cracked wheat breads, whole-grain breakfast cereals, fresh fruits and vegetables, and almonds. The almond is of particular benefit because it is high in fiber and is the only nut that is alkaline in nature. These nuts may be eaten either raw (preferably two to four each day for at least three days a week), when baking, or in other food preparations.

COMMENT: The purpose of the aforementioned diets, cathartics and cleansing methods can be expressed in one word, DETOXIFICATION. These cover only some of the available options that I have presented to my patients. Some choices are more effective than others for different individuals. Selecting the most effective ones can only be determined by the attending physician and the patient.

Fume and Steam Baths

One of the oldest forms of body rejuvenation, cleansing, and stimulation of the skin is the ancient fume or steam bath. The purpose behind taking this form of hydrotherapy (if available) is to open the pores in order to aid the removal of toxins through the sweat glands of the skin. If the skin is extremely sensitive and almost tissue-thin, as often occurs in severe exfoliative psoriasis, I do not recommend steam. Fortunately, these very extreme cases are rare. This type of hydrotherapy can be undertaken either by purchasing a home unit or using those found at Spas or Health Clubs.

CAUTION: *If a patient suffers from a heart problem, high blood pressure, or from any other questionable systemic condition, subjecting him or her to steam, a steam room, or a steam cabinet is NOT advised.*

Even if there is no reason to expect an adverse reaction to steam, I still advise that an attendant be on hand in order to apply cool towels to the head and neck in case the patient becomes overheated while in a steam cabinet. The cabinet encloses the whole body, but leaves the head exposed to permit sufficient oxygen intake. The patient sits in this specially made unit while steam is generated and engulfs the entire body.

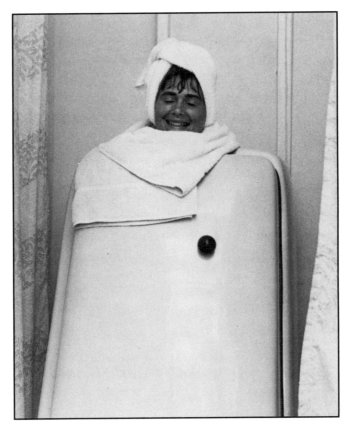

Fig. 5-6
A steam cabinet in use.

For psoriatic conditions, Cayce advised that a mixture of one tablespoon of witch hazel in half a pint of water be placed in the reservoir of the steam cabinet. The average time limit for remaining in a steam cabinet is approximately twenty to thirty minutes. This may vary five minutes either way. It is important to learn how much steam a patient can tolerate without any adverse effects. It is best to shower down after having a steam or fume bath with plain, warm water. Using soap is avoided, for this will tend to clog the pores of the skin again.

NOTE: A large amount of body fluids is lost when having a steam or fume bath. Each person has a different tolerance and reaction to this loss of fluid. If the loss becomes excessive, the reaction is similar to that of a person suffering from heat prostration and the same treatment is called for. The classic signs are fainting, dizziness and weakness. It is vital to replace the salt lost from the tissue cells. Therefore, I make sure my patients drink a glass of water to which a pinch of salt has been added both *before* and *after* having a steam bath, as well as one or two glasses of pure water while taking the steam. In order to prevent any loss of potassium and calcium, it is best that they eat foods rich in these minerals, again both *before* and *after* this form of therapy, to avoid any depletion.

I can't help but recall the adverse reaction one of my former patients experienced from loss of salt. After traveling on an extremely hot day in a non-airconditioned bus, and feeling totally exhausted, she went for a scheduled steam bath. While in the steam cabinet, she felt faint and weak. The attendant in charge immediately removed her from the cabinet and called to inform me of her reaction. I suggested that he give her a glass of water to which a quarter-teaspoon of salt had been added. Upon drinking the water, she found that her faintness and weakness disappeared almost instantaneously. This is akin to the experience of athletes who take salt tablets on hot days in order to replace any salt they might lose through profuse sweating.

Saffron Tea or Saffron Water and Steam Baths

Another measure I suggest to my patients that will help derive the greatest benefit from steam is to drink a cup of saffron tea or a 6-8 oz. glass of saffron water about 1/2 to 1 hour before taking the steam bath. The steam will open the pores of the skin and the saffron tea or water will work its way right through the skin carrying toxins along with it, thus aiding the internal cleansing process. I consider this a most valued procedure to follow if the patient has access to a steam bath. Both Saffron Tea and Saffron Water are covered in Chapter 7, "Herb Teas".

The precautions are basically the same as for Epsom Salts baths. No cardiovascular case should have a steam or fume bath, and there should always be an attendant on hand to water down and watch the patient's reaction. If the skin is too sensitive with the addition of witch hazel, plain steam may be all that can be used in the beginning. I *do not* recommend Sauna baths be taken in cases of psoriasis or eczema.

Each patient must judge what he or she can or cannot tolerate. I advise all who inquire to check with their own doctor before attempting the fume or steam bath. Effective as they are, to some they may be harmful.

Exercise

Exercise is a vital part of the regimen for clearing psoriasis. It stimulates the internal structures of the body, increases circulation, activates the glands, oxygenates the blood, opens the pores, pumps the lymph, and filters the blood through the liver and kidneys.

Exercising, especially in the open air, provides untold benefits. I encourage my patients to participate in *non-contact* sports such as tennis, badminton, golf, jogging (moderately), walking, and swimming. Contact sports should be avoided because psoriatics have a sensitive dermal layer of the skin. If you may recall, it is often noted that the disease first appears after there is a bruise to the skin.

Bicycling, either outdoors or on a stationary home unit, rowing and low-impact aerobics, at home or in a health club, are additional forms of exercise that are beneficial to the psoriatic and should be done on a regular basis, two or three times a week. Stretching exercises also aid the body in eliminating waste matter more effectively, but for those who have psoriasis, it must be remembered that stretching may also traumatize the sensitive layers of the skin; therefore, this should be done gently and in moderation. Social dancing stimulates all internal structures, and consequently also helps in the cleansing process.

The most effective type of walking is "brisk" walking, out of doors, rain or shine. Rhythmic breathing while walking doubles its effectiveness. This is accomplished by inhaling for six counts, holding your breath for six counts, and then exhaling for six counts. Doing this will help to develop a pattern in your daily walking routine. If possible, set a specific time for walking each day and never walk to the point of exhaustion. When walking, the mind should be free of any nagging problems, or the desired benefits will be lost in the murk and mire of destructive thinking.

It has been suggested that if you want to prevent a heart attack, you should get yourself a dog. Why? Because you will have to walk your dog *regularly*. Most of us neglect to do any walking, especially in the evening, because we prefer to watch television. Owning a dog forces us out of this sedentary habit.

I can personally vouch for this advice, for there have been many instances when, after a full day of seeing patients, the last thing I wanted to do was walk my dog, Shane. But he would look up at me with soulful eyes as if to say, "O.K., now it's time to take care of *me*." I would drag myself out of my chair to get his leash, stagger through the door, and begin our walk. Before long, a new consciousness of well-being would come over me. Where did the tiredness disappear to, and where did my renewed energy come from? Perhaps it came from the production of endorphines, a benefit recently discovered by the jogging set. Whatever the reason, once I started walking, I felt different, oxygenated, and alert. I realized suddenly that it was not I who had been taking care of Shane...it was he who was taking care of me!

Swimming has long been recognized as a most beneficial sport and physical activity, provided that the water you swim in is free of pollution. It is so effective because it exercises every muscle, joint and ligament of the body. It also aids respiration, circulation, and flexibility, which is one of the most important elements in warding off old age and its typical stiffness. Swimming in clear water, especially ocean water, cleanses and stimulates the skin, thereby helping to wash away toxins. The benefits are too numerous to mention. Make swimming a part of your life, and vigor and vitality will accompany you wherever you go. An aura of youthfulness will surround you—and if you radiate health, health will most surely accompany you all the days of your life.

FIND THE TIME TO EXERCISE!...or nature will eventually provide you with nothing but time, flat on your back.

Toxins

Since toxic buildup is what actually causes psoriasis, it will do no harm for the psoriatic to learn about the meaning of the word "toxin." If nothing else, the patient will at least be able to identify the enemy.

To begin with, a toxin is a poisonous substance derived from animal or vegetable cells. When toxins invade the bloodstream, the result is *toxemia*, a condition in which the blood contains an overabundance of poisons. Toxins are produced by body cells or by the growth of microorganisms which cause a general infection, whereby the blood contains toxins but not bacteria. When the buildup becomes too much for the body's natural defense mechanism to handle, the patient is considered *toxic*. Symptoms such as tiredness, malaise, lack of energy, etc., and often halitosis (bad breath), are common signs of toxicity.

Why is it important for the psoriatic to understand what toxemia is? Pottenger states that "in all cases of toxemia, and particularly those of acute toxemia, we find a tendency to *sluggishness of action in the gastrointestinal tract*"[6] [Emphasis added].

Obviously, when this "sluggishness" occurs there is a greater tendency for re-absorbing toxic elements through the walls of both the small and large intestines. It is my contention that this is the major cause of most degenerative, debilitating diseases, as well as various skin conditions, including psoriasis.

Improved Bathroom Facilities

Since the turn of this century, man's life span has doubled. Most of us presume that this is due to advances in medical technology, wonder drugs, surgical procedures, etc. Undoubtedly, these have contributed greatly to man's longevity. Seldom recognized, however, is the role that improved sanitary conditions play, especially the advent of indoor plumbing. A new era of health and longevity began when toilet facilities within the home came upon the scene. Today, such accommodations are taken for granted, especially among young people. In years gone by, and not too long ago at that, the "outhouse" was recognized as the cubicle of privacy. As it was located at least several yards away from the main house, it involved extra effort, especially in the dead of winter. The tendency was to wait, avoiding evacuation until absolutely necessary. On occasion, it would be days before one relieved himself. This naturally caused a backup pressure of fecal matter which often was allowed to reach a point of *autointoxication*, and unquestionably acted as a precursor of many systemic diseases. Evidence of this is found in comparing our present-day life span of eighty years or so with the average of about forty years at the turn of the century. It is no longer necessary to retain all the poisons and waste matter because of uncomfortable, inconvenient toilet facilities, for indoor plumbing provides relief but a few steps away in the comfort of your own home.

The "Glut" Response

Toxins form not only from substances known to be detrimental to the body but from those that may become toxic if overindulged in. Ordinarily such substances, notably food items, may not have a deleterious effect, but because of an insatiable desire for a particular food, some people have a tendency to gorge themselves. This causes what I call a "glut" response. In these cases, a chemical imbalance is bound to occur, and the body will respond by producing skin conditions, allergic reactions, glandular dysfunctions, and a myriad of other ailments.

Here is one situation where I must ardently disagree with the advice of that great lady of stage and screen, Mae West, who once said, "Listen, honey, too much of a good thing...can be wonderful!"

Thoughts and Toxins

As previously emphasized, clearing the body of accumulated toxins is of the utmost importance. Just as significant, however, is the maintenance of a healthy mental attitude. Have no doubt about it—*negative, destructive thoughts also produce acidic toxins that can do still more harm to an already polluted system.*

For instance, one cannot have continued feelings of hatred without developing stomach or liver problems. Negative emotions such as uncontrollable anger or jealousy can cause digestive or heart disorders. Animosity and worrying can only lead to further distressful systemic conditions.

Thoughts most assuredly affect the internal environment of the body. This is now fully accepted and recognized by the scientific community.

One should learn to recognize and appreciate the cheerful aspects of life and avoid involving oneself with negative situations and personalities, referred to in modern parlance as "real downers"!

A sunny, smiling countenance goes a long way, not only for yourself but for those around you. This important subject matter is further discussed in my chapter, "The Emotional Factor."

The bottom line then is to rid the body of toxins that have accumulated over a long period of time and avoid reintroducing those same toxic elements to the system. Learn to recognize the pollutants, usually certain foods, and avoid them at all costs.

We start the entire process with INTERNAL CLEANSING as we would take a bath or shower before dressing up in a new suit of clothes; the difference here being that the bath or shower is done on the inside and the new suit will be realized in time as a new, revitalized beautiful skin.

REFERENCES

(Chapter 5—Internal Cleansing)

1. Frederick D. Lansford Jr., M.D., "Commentary on Psoriasis" in *Physician's Reference Notebook*, ed. by William A. McGarey, M.D., (Virginia Beach, VA, The A.R.E. Press, Sept. 1968 Ed. 1) p. 189.
2. Francis M. Pottenger, M.D., *Symptoms of Visceral Disease*, ed. 7, (St. Louis, 1953, The C.V. Mosby Co.) p. 272. Reprinted by permission.
3. Edgar Cayce Reference # 2002-1, (Virginia Beach, VA, The Edgar Cayce Foundation, copyright 1971). Reprinted by permission.
4. Henry G. Bieler, M.D., *Food Is Your Best Medicine*, (New York, NY, copyright 1973, Random House, Inc.) pp. 42-43. Reprinted by permission.
5. Charles Best, M.D., and Norman Taylor, M.D., *The Living Body*, (New York, NY, Henry Holt & Co., copyright 1952, ed. 3), p. 381.
6. Pottenger, p. 280.

Chapter 6

Diet and Nutrition

(Basics)

In the management and control of psoriasis, the significance of an effective diet has been questioned for as long as the disease has been researched. The fact is that as early as 1932, the beneficial effects that diet has on psoriasis were clearly demonstrated by Jay F. Schamberg, M.D., a former professor of dermatology at the University of Pennsylvania. His work, however, was largely overlooked in this endeavor and seemed to simply fade into oblivion. More on his works, and others even earlier, will be discussed in the latter part of this chapter.

For many patients, this controversial issue has caused much confusion and bewilderment. Since authorities constantly contradict each other, patients are usually left in a dietary dilemma. In most cases, they would be eager to follow a nutritional program if one were available to them. Should a physician mention diet, it is usually only in a cursory manner or totally dismissed as having little or no effect in alleviating this disease. It is in this area that I feel the scientific community should become more cognizant of its intrinsic value. My research and treatment have proven to me beyond question, that *DIET not only plays a distinctive role, but is indeed the most important factor in healing psoriasis.* Besides being the very foundation of the recommended therapy, it is also the key factor in preventing its recurrence.

In all the years that I have been treating psoriasis cases, I have never achieved successful results if the diet was not followed at least to a reasonable degree. Other recommended measures are valuable aids and most certainly assist in hastening positive results in healing this skin disorder. However, without the underlying common denominator of proper diet, the effort is fruitless. If this statement sounds like an exaggerated claim, I can assure you it is not. A psoriatic must fully accept and understand that the consumption as well as avoidance of certain foods is *vital* to his or her recovery from this dermatological problem. If a patient is not willing to accept this as fact, it may be necessary to revert back to the more orthodox forms of therapy rather than the alternative route presented herein.

I do not wish to mislead my readers into believing that the recommended measures, including the prescribed diet, guarantee success. There are a variety of reasons for failures. In many cases, however, those who did not receive beneficial results were patients who refused to alter their dietary habits—or—if they did, did not do so for a long enough period of time. When I begin to sense this attitude, usually after a few visits, I discourage them from continuing. My efforts are reserved for those who are at least willing to give this more natural approach time and an opportunity to work. One is rarely successful when they say that they will try to go on the diet for a few weeks. Most seem to forget that it took considerable time to pollute every tissue cell of the body before the poisons bulged through their skin in the form of psoriasis. Yet, once the cleansing process takes effect, it is amazing how often the body quickly responds in a matter of months, sometimes weeks. The most devastating lesions simply seem to dry up and disappear once the body is given the proper tools to work with.

Granted, there are some who developed psoriatic lesions and experienced a complete remission of the disease for unknown reasons. There are also those who simply rubbed salves or ointments on their skin and achieved similar results. Needless to say, these cases do not have to be concerned with extensive therapies or diets. However, it would be well for them to remember that they are prone to the disease if only to a minor degree and should, therefore, cultivate and develop an awareness of which foods are beneficial to them as well as those that are not.

The psoriatics that I am most concerned with are those who are chronically plagued with the disease, those who have sought relief for many years—some, most of their lives. They reach an impenetrable barrier when seeking explanations as to its cause and a therapy that is relatively risk-free, successful and lasting. I reach out to these sufferers and irrevocably declare that there are answers to their problem, in both cause and management; the most important of which is found in *their daily diet.*

When Cayce was asked if there was an absolute cure for psoriasis, his answer was straight and to the point:

"MOST OF THIS IS FOUND IN DIET. THERE IS A CURE. IT REQUIRES PATIENCE, PERSISTENCE—AND—RIGHT THINKING ALSO."

This discourse (2455-2), in my estimation, is the most profound of all the Cayce works that pertain to psoriasis. In a few brief passages, he gives us the clue; the direction, if you will, of freeing oneself of an enigma that has plagued mankind for centuries. "The itch for which there is no cure" can even be found in Biblical teachings. It very well could be that the "itch" they refer to was psoriasis. Cayce provided us with an answer; it was my task to prove it!

Thankfully, there presently is a resurgence of interest in nutrition. Today, more than ever before, the public recognizes the role that nutritious foods play in maintaining a general state of well-being. It can no longer be ignored or even taken lightly, as is evidenced in recent cancer research. We are being forced to return to nature and natural foods for sustenance. The trick is to prevent further pollution of our soil and water in order to insure proper elements are supplied to our growing crops. Let us remember, however, that the final chapter on diet and nutrition has not yet been written. New findings replace old "facts" every day.

Therefore, the idea of an illness such as psoriasis responding favorably to changes in diet is no longer remote. Has it not been said for ages that we are mentally what we think and physically what we eat? This holds true particularly in the case of psoriatics. Fortunately, as human beings, we have the power to control both to a large extent.

THE ACID-ALKALINE BALANCE

What is it about diet that is so vital to the psoriatic? It is the importance of maintaining the proper Acid/Alkaline (Base) Balance of the body chemistry. Although this subject was briefly touched upon in an earlier chapter it is of such value that it warrants discussing again in more detail.

Nature *demands* that the body remain more on the Alkaline side rather than on the Acid side for the preservation of good health. The body becomes more resistant to all types of disease and physical ailments when engulfed in this internal chemical atmosphere. Arthritic joints are greatly relieved, colds and congestion are counteracted, skin problems diminish, and internal organs become less burdened.[1]

It must not be assumed that acids are not important, for they most certainly are, but in their proper proportion.

The 80%/20% Food Ratio

One's blood should always be slightly alkaline, with a pH of 7.3 to 7.5, in chemical reaction in order to maintain the optimum in general health and immunity.[2] This is primarily maintained by the body's natural "lines of defense" and most certainly influenced by the foods ingested and from one's emotional makeup.

In later chapters we will explore the effects generated by destructive thoughts and negative emotions. It is the food intake and tremendous influence it has on the psoriatic that we are most concerned with in this section.

The psoriatic, psoriatic arthritic and eczema patient should keep before his mind's eye the ratio of "80%/20%" at all times! This means that *THE DAILY DIET SHOULD CONSIST OF 80% ALKALINE-FORMING FOODS AND 20% ACID-FORMING FOODS*—or—to state it more simply, many more alkaline forming foods should be consumed than acid formers.

With most of us, our eating habits are just the opposite. We fill ourselves with acid-forming foods which produce a hyperacidic condition and then wonder why our joints are stiff in the morning, find ourselves more susceptible to colds, and develop skin blemishes, especially as we get older. This is because the acids become overabundant in the body and the cells cry out for relief. It is nothing less than amazing to see how quickly a patient responds, in a positive way, when the shift from acidity to alkalinity takes place. Joints become more flexible and less painful, colds and congestion, as well as some allergies often clear up, and the skin takes on a healthier glow with many blemishes disappearing. Results are lasting if a patient does not revert back to his or her previous eating habits after being relieved of these conditions.

Obviously, it becomes mandatory that a patient learn which foods are Alkaline and which are Acid, as well as those that should be avoided altogether, such as the Nightshades and most saturated fats and sweets.

There have been occasions when, unknowingly, some of my patients gradually lost track of maintaining the 80%/20% ratio of foods and found themselves eating more of the 20% Acid-Formers than they should simply because they were listed as "Allowed" foods. Lesions gradually began to resurface without the patient realizing why. Once they were made aware of the reason for this shift to the Acid side, their diet was altered to include more AlkalineFormers than Acid-Formers. As a result, the lesions slowly began to retract.

Additionally, specific habits and physical activities have an influence on Acid/Alkaline reactions in the body. Recognizing those that are beneficial or harmful is of the utmost importance. This subject matter will be covered in more detail as we proceed.

ALKALINE FORMERS vs. ACID FORMERS

Modern nutritionists agree that, in general, fruits are the primary *cleansers* of the body, while vegetables are considered to be the *builders*.

ALKALINE FORMERS

ALKALINE-FORMING FOODS—(80% of the Daily Diet)—are the more "watery" type fruits, vegetables, and their juices. Because these foods are broken down more easily by the body, they are more readily digested.

MOST FRUITS are Alkaline-Formers (Reacting) within the body, with the exception of only five which are Acid-Forming. They are: Cranberries, Currants, Large Prunes, Plums and Blueberries. The benefits and nutrition derived from fresh fruits, in general, far outweigh the minor acidic content of these few exceptions. Consequently, I therefore usually advise my patients to eat fresh fruits often without being overly concerned about their Acid/Alkaline content, as long as it is not overdone or they do not cause an adverse reaction. Consuming too much Fruit or Fruit Juice can induce elevated triglycerides because excess fruit sugars can be retained in the body tissues as stored fat.

COMMENT: In nutritional terms, fruits are divided into three categories: Acid, Sub-Acid and Sweet. The reader, however, should not be confused with these terms and regard them as Acid-Forming, for, in fact, most so-called "Acid" fruits are actually Alkaline-Reacting in the body.

THE FOLLOWING FRUITS SHOULD BE ACCORDED SPECIAL ATTENTION:

- *STRAWBERRIES, CITRUS FRUIT* and *CITRUS JUICES* should be *avoided* in cases of Psoriatic Arthritis or if there is a Hypersensitive reaction. In addition, *AVOCADO* should be avoided if a patient has Gout.

- *RAW APPLES, MELONS* and *BANANAS should not* be combined with other foods, i.e. in fruit salads, cereals, etc., or as part of a regular meal such as an appetizer or dessert. These fruits, however, may be eaten *separately* as a snack or between meals. In other words, "Eat Them Alone or Leave Them Alone."

- *CITRUS FRUITS*—Namely: Oranges, Grapefruit, Lemons, Limes, Kumquat, Tangerines, Mandarins, Pomelo, Pummelo, Shaddock, Tangelo, and Citrangedin and their JUICES *should not be combined* with Whole-Grains, Dairy Products or any White Flour Product, i.e. Cereals, Breads, Muffins, Pancakes, Milk, Eggs, Butter, Yogurt, Cheese, etc. The only exception regarding the above is for particularly active children and for other individuals whose daily activities require them to expend a great deal of energy. These people may combine Citrus Fruits and Juices with Whole-Grain Products, (no White Flour Products) provided there are no adverse reactions. If the skin becomes hypersensitive or irritated from eating too many Citrus Fruits, I recommend eliminating or consuming less of them, in favor of Non-Citrus Fruits.

MOST VEGETABLES are also Alkaline-Formers (Reacting) within the body, except for the following, which are Acid-Forming. They are: Legumes (Dried Beans and Peas; Kidney, Pinto, Black and Navy Beans; Black-Eyed, Split and Chick Peas)—Lentils—and the following vegetables, Mature Corn (Large Kernels), Dried Corn, Rhubarb, Winter Squash (Hubbard, Acorn, Butternut), and Brussel Sprouts. Although these vegetables are Acid-Reacting they may still be consumed, but in smaller quantities. It is advisable to eat three vegetables that grow above the ground, i.e. Lettuce, Celery, Spinach, Broccoli, etc., to one that grows below the ground, i.e. Carrots, Beets, Sweet Potatoes, Onions, etc.—[A more detailed chart of ABOVE and BELOW GROUND VEGETABLES may be found in Appendix A.] It should be noted that consuming an overabundance of any one vegetable, fruit or juice that may be high in vitamins which are naturally stored in the body, Vitamins A, D, E & K, may trigger an adverse reaction, therefore, moderation should be exercised.

SUGGESTION: More vitamins and minerals are assimilated by drinking freshly-made vegetable juice to which one packet of Unflavored Gelatin has been added. In order to obtain the maximum benefit, this juice should be consumed within ten minutes after being prepared.

BEWARE—THE NIGHTSHADES!—It would be well for all psoriatic and eczema patients to familiarize themselves with the term NIGHTSHADE. This represents a family of plants that they should *totally AVOID* regardless of their Acid/Alkaline reaction. The Nightshades are: Tomatoes, Tobacco, Eggplant, White Potatoes, Peppers and Paprika. This subject matter will be covered further in this chapter. Suffice it here to simply list them for the sake of recognition.

THE FOLLOWING MEASURES ALSO HELP TO INCREASE ALKALINITY IN THE BODY AND SHOULD THEREFORE BE INCORPORATED IN ONE'S DIET AND LIFE-STYLE:

- Adding Granular Lecithin, an Alkaline Food Supplement, to Foods and Beverages—[Lecithin will be covered in more detail later in this Chapter]

- Freshly-squeezed Lemon Juice in a cup of Hot or Cold Water—Many patients have found this to be a good substitute for Hot Tea or Coffee. Not only does it help maintain the alkalinity but aids the internal cleansing process.

- Consuming nutritious Fruit Juices such as : Grape, Pear, Papaya, Apricot, Guava, Mango and Pineapple

- Combining Grapefruit or Orange Juice (4 parts) with Fresh Lemon or Lime Juice (1 part)

- Fresh or Stewed Fruits

- Consuming Vegetable Juices extracted from Raw Carrots, Celery, Beets, Parsley, Romaine Lettuce and Spinach—Raw Onions are particularly cleansing

- Exercising and Physical Activities, especially out-of-doors

- Having a bowel evacuation at least once or twice a day

- Positive Emotions such as: Self-Confidence, A Loving Nature, A Sense of Humor, Laughter, The Ability to Forgive, etc.

- Three to Five Drops of Glyco-Thymoline in a glass of pure water, before retiring, 5 days per week. [This Alkaline-Cleansing Solution will be covered further in this chapter.]

ACID-FORMERS

ACID-FORMING FOODS (20% of the Daily Diet) are the heavier, more solid foods (Proteins, Starches, Sugars, Fats and Oils). Combinations of these foods, especially when consumed in large quantities, build up the acid content of the blood and consequently aggravate a psoriatic condition. Meats, Grains, Cheese, Sugars, Potatoes, Dry Peas and Beans, Oils, Butter, Cream and Prepared Meats (Frankfurters, Salami, Bologna, etc.) are the most common Acid-Formers. These foods require the digestive organs to produce more acids in order to break them down for absorption. In this case, what remains is called an ACID ASH. Depending on the type of food consumed, the body is left with either an ACID ASH or an ALKALINE ASH. The ideal chemical reaction is one that tends toward an ALKALINE ASH; thus the reasoning behind the 80% Alkaline—20% Acid Food intake. Acid-Forming Foods, although a relatively small percentage of the daily diet, are nevertheless, *vital* to the body's growth, repair and development.

THE MEASURES BELOW ALSO TEND TO INCREASE ACIDITY IN THE BODY AND SHOULD THEREFORE BE AVOIDED AS MUCH AS POSSIBLE:

- Combining too many Acid-Forming Foods at the same meal—For example: Starches with Sweets—Proteins and Meats—Meats or Fats with Sugars—too many Starchy Foods [A list of Proteins and Starches may be found in Appendix A]

- Consuming Cane Sugar and any product made from Cane Sugar

- Most types of Vinegar, especially wine vinegar and white (grain) vinegar

- Eating foods that contain large amounts of Preservatives, Artificial Flavorings, Colorings and Additives

- Alcoholic Beverages

- Smoking

- Drug Abuse

- Constipation

- Inactivity—both Mental or Physical

- Negative Emotions such as: Insecurity, Fearfulness, Worry, Over-Anxiety, Jealousy, Resentment, Feelings of Inferiority, and Destructive Thoughts in general

The Effect Toxemia Has on the Acid/Alkaline (Base) Balance

I ask my readers to carefully ponder the following scientific fact revealed in Francis M. Pottenger's, *Symptoms of Visceral Disease*. It clearly defines the effect that toxemia (poisons in the blood) has on the Acid/Alkaline chemistry of the body's tissues:

"When toxemia is prolonged, a loss of body bases occurs which results in a shifting of the acid/alkali balance of the tissues toward the acid side. This has an important bearing on the production and prolongation of toxic symptoms. This condition calls for the administration of alkalis, either in the form of alkaline foods or alkaline salts. This is more marked in some diseases than in others."[3]

Psoriasis is one of those diseases in which there is a decided shift in the body chemistry to the acid side. A psoriasis patient, therefore, must be *aware* of the significance of maintaining a proper balance and he or she must be willing to follow the suggested diet and regimen for as long as necessary.

Glyco-Thymoline

Glyco-Thymoline, which was previously mentioned in the Chapter, "Internal Cleansing" is an intestinal antiseptic and is alkaline in nature. This substance, when taken internally (4 or 5 drops in a glass of water before retiring, 5 days per week), is beneficial to the psoriatic, psoriatic arthritic and eczema sufferer, in that it promotes alkalinity and cleanses the digestive tract which, in turn, reduces toxemia.

In some cases, Glyco-Thymoline, when externally applied full strength on small, affected areas, has proven to be quite soothing in relieving severe itching (Pruritus).

Although this is a non-prescription item (a mouth wash), if taken internally, it must first be approved by an M.D. or Osteopath. If this product is unavailable in a local drugstore, my patients may obtain it from either Home Health Products, Inc., or The Heritage Store, Inc., both located in Virginia Beach, VA. [See Appendix C.]

Lecithin

I suggest that all of my psoriasis patients take Lecithin regularly. Derived primarily from soybeans, Lecithin, rich in non-animal proteins and highly alkaline, has been considered by many nutritionists to be a fat emulsifier. In simple terms, it prevents blood fat (Cholesterol) from accumulating in the arteries by keeping it in suspension. Arteriosclerosis develops from accumulations of fat deposits on the arterial walls. It is believed that Lecithin helps to prevent this from happening. Contrary to this concept, however, the value of Lecithin is held in dispute, according to an article which appeared in the October 1989 Tufts University Newsletter (Vol. 7, No. 8). Their report states that studies conducted since 1943 indicate that Lecithin has no effect in reducing blood cholesterol levels and that claims of its beneficial aspects have no basis in fact.

Other studies, however, do recognize Lecithin as a beneficial health measure, including the influence it has on thought processes. German scientists state: "No phosphoric acid—no brain." Phosphorus, in the form of phosphoric acid is found in Lecithin and is essential in human physiology, especially in brain and nerve tissue. Lecithin has been used in therapeutic doses for patients suffering from degenerative diseases, such as scleroderma and rheumatoid arthritis, as well as diseases with neurological involvement, such as multiple sclerosis (MS) or amyotrophic lateral sclerosis (ALS).

Lecithin and Psoriasis

In her book, *Let's Get Well*, Adelle Davis refers to psoriasis as an "eczema-like skin condition which appears to result from faulty utilization of fats."[4] This world-renowned nutritionist reports that when 254 psoriasis patients were given 4 to 8 tablespoons of Lecithin daily, no new eruptions occurred after the first week and the most severe cases recovered within five months. She also states that people with this abnormality usually have excessive amounts of cholesterol in their skin and blood. By the time their blood cholesterol is reduced to normal, their psoriasis is no longer evident. Even though she reports these findings, I have personally found with my patients that those with severe psoriasis, more often than not, had perfectly normal blood pictures, and in some cases, a surprisingly *low* cholesterol count. I make this comparison only to show that the blood picture is not necessarily a key factor in evaluating psoriasis. A blood test, however, known as an SMA-12 or an SMA-24, along with a urinalysis, may show other abnormalities which a physician should be aware of.

In addition to Lecithin being harmless, non-habit forming, alkaline, and an aid to digestion, there is another important benefit, especially to the psoriatic; it has a decided effect on bowel evacuation. I have found that Lecithin acts as an excellent, natural laxative.

I recommend my patients take 1 Tablespoon of granular Lecithin three times a day, 5 days a week. It makes no difference how it is consumed, therefore, it may be added to water, juice, sprinkled over a salad or cereal. Once a patient's skin is clear, I recommend that the Lecithin intake is reduced to 1 Tablespoon a day, five days a week.

Lecithin is now readily available in any well supplied health food store, drug store or supermarket and comes in three forms: liquid, tablet or granular. I prefer granules because the phosphatide content is highest in this form. It is the phosphatide content of Lecithin that emulsifies the blood fat. Admittedly, the liquid capsule form is more convenient and easier to swallow. However, it takes nine capsules (1200 mg. each) to equal the amount of phosphatides found in one level tablespoon of Lecithin granules. It should be noted, however, that like all over-the-counter substances, Lecithin should not be abused by overuse for, in this case, it may interfere with calcium absorption.

A Case in Point

As I stated previously, the therapeutic effects of Lecithin are far-reaching and sometimes quite surprising. Once at a dinner party, I happened to sit next to a dear friend and noticed how unusually "picky" she was regarding the foods that were served. I had never noticed her being so choosy about the foods she ate in the past, for she always seemed able to enjoy anything and everything. When I inquired why she was particularly selective about her foods, she related that in the past few months she was unable to eat foods that contained fat, particularly milk and animal fats. The reactions of eating these foods produced devastating discomfort in the form of welts, throat constriction and skin eruptions. There seemed to be no logical explanation for this sudden change in food reactions. I suggested that she consider taking Lecithin daily. Even though she was not familiar with this product, she agreed to try it since it was a natural substance.

When next I met her at another dinner party, she was able to eat anything that was placed before her with no adverse reactions! She informed me that after beginning to take Lecithin, her difficulty with digesting fats stopped almost immediately. Since then, she continues to take Lecithin regularly, remains free of the problem, and attributes her recovery entirely to it.

It must not be assumed that everyone will have the same reaction from taking Lecithin. In this particular case, however, the results were so dramatic that I felt it warranted comment.

Atmospheric Influence on the Acid/Alkaline Balance

It is common knowledge that most psoriatic conditions usually improve during the summer and get worse in the winter. During the colder months, home-heating units reduce the humidity in the air and subsequently, dry out the skin. A humidifier usually corrects this situation. In summer, because less clothing is worn, beneficial sunrays are allowed to penetrate the skin which bring about a healing influence. In addition, much more water is normally consumed during the summer months which aids the internal cleansing process.

It was extremely interesting for me to come across a series of charts by S.W. Tromp that compared *physiological processes* in the body with *observed seasonal changes*. In his book, *How Atmospheric Conditions Affect Your Health*,[5] author, Michel Gauguelin, a science writer and French researcher in Psychology and Statistics at the Sorbonne, presents these charts which show the effects that seasons have on the acid/alkaline contents of the gastrointestinal tract. Among the myriad of functions listed was the fact that *Gastro-acidity increases in the winter and is low in the summer; while Gastro-alkalinity is high in the summer and low in the winter*. This, in itself, adds credence to the possible link of acid/alkaline balance relative to psoriasis.

Avoiding the Nightshades

As mentioned earlier in this chapter, a psoriatic must become well-acquainted with the term, NIGHTSHADE, for it denotes a group of the most undesirable substances that should be avoided. Nightshade, as some of my readers may know, is a deadly poison (atropa belladonna). Most people recognize this simply as "Belladonna" which is used only for medicinal purposes.

Unprecedented research has been conducted by Norman F. Childers, Ph.D., formerly of the Agricultural Department of Rutgers University, who is presently continuing his work at the University of Florida, Institute of Food and Agricultural Sciences at Gainesville, Florida. He has compiled overwhelming evidence that the nightshades have a most deleterious effect on people afflicted with arthritis and may even be a basic cause. Psoriasis and arthritis, in my opinion, are closely allied diseases because I have found quite often that they both respond favorably to the regimen contained herein. In a later chapter, "The Arthritic Connection," this is covered in more detail.

[NOTE: Dr. Norman F. Childers' book, *Arthritis—Childers' Diet To Stop It!* may be ordered from Horticultural Publications, 3906 N.W. 31 Place, Gainesville, Florida 32606. Phone: (904) 372-5077.]

THE NIGHTSHADES:

1. Tomatoes (and their derivatives)

2. Tobacco

3. Eggplant

4. White Potatoes

5. Peppers (except the seasoning, Black Pepper)

6. Paprika

TOMATOES—During my years of research, I have personally observed that many of my psoriatic patients absolutely "loved" tomatoes. Prior to being aware of Dr. Childers' findings, I noticed how detrimental tomatoes were to my patients and consequently eliminated them from their diet. As soon as I did, there was a slow, but marked improvement in their condition. While corresponding with Dr. Childers, he informed me that he too achieved similar results. Tomatoes, therefore, and their derivatives (juice, ketchup, sauces, etc.) rank highest in foods to *avoid*.

TOBACCO—Since tobacco is also a nightshade, smoking should be completely avoided or at least greatly curtailed.Cigarette smoking poisons the respiratory system, contracts small blood vessels that can lead to heart disease, and among other factors, has an acidic effect on the body. For those who insist upon smoking, however, and are unable to break this habit, they should try to limit themselves to only a few cigarettes per day.

WHITE POTATOES—The pulp as well as the skin of the white potato should be avoided. Research conducted at Cornell University in 1987 indicates that the skin of white potatoes contain toxic substances known as glycoalkaloids. Although the average person may be immune, this substance can adversely affect sensitive individuals to an alarming degree. In addition, Dr. Childers, from the University of Florida, also concludes that the skins contain the highest amount of toxins. Because of the fact that Yams or Sweet Potatoes are considered to be part of the "Morning-glory" family of plants and are not Nightshades, they, as well as their skins, are permitted as long as they are baked, boiled or steamed and not fried.

This is one area that conflicts with Cayce for he highly recommended eating the skins of potatoes but not the pulp for the general public. We must remember, however, that we are dealing with psoriasis. What may not affect the average person can have a most serious effect on a psoriatic; thus, the reason for my suggesting that my patients abstain from eating white potato skins as well as the pulp.

EGGPLANT, PEPPERS and PAPRIKA—These foods should not be consumed, again, because of the highly toxic effect they have on the psoriatic. One of my patients, in particular, attributed the great improvement in his condition due to the elimination of two favorite foods from his diet— eggplant and peppers. Hot, spicy foods, especially those made from nightshades, are to be totally avoided. I am convinced that the high incidence of psoriasis in India is largely due to the country's hot, spicy diet.

Pizza—America's Favorite Food

It is well known that Americans love pizza. It has become more American than Mom's apple pie, and is gaining in popularity in all corners of the earth. To the psoriatic, however, it is one of the worst food items that they can consume. Practically all of the ingredients that comprise a pizza contribute to an over-acidic condition. For instance, it's base is usually made with white flour, tomato sauce (a nightshade) is spread on top of this, followed by a thick layer of cheese. Peppers, also a nightshade, are a favorite pizza topping as well as sausage, pepperoni, hot spices and condiments. Put them all together and they spell "HELL" to the psoriatic.

One patient related a story to me that is worth retelling. She was admitted into one of the major dermatological centers in New York City for a three-week stay in which PUVA therapy was her entire daily regimen. At the end of this period and to the tune of $20,000, she left the hospital with clear skin. It took exactly *one day* for the lesions to return in full bloom. As I notated her case history, I learned that diet, in general, was never a subject discussed at the center. In fact, she further related that if patients showed an interest in diet, their queries were simply made light of with the insinuation that it was of no consequence. You can imagine my concern when she informed me that a party was held for all the psoriatics in her particular group at the end of her hospital stay. What kind of party?... A PIZZA party!

Metaphorically speaking: Eat pizza and you will soon resemble one. If I have not been convincing enough, I urge my readers to view the case of Ms. A.M. located in the color portfolio section. As inconceivable as it may seem, her daily diet consisted of eating pizza every day, and practically no other foods. In her case, desperation forced her to seek alternative routes and she found herself on my doorstep in April 1987. Needless to say, I immediately eliminated pizza from her diet and placed her on the prescribed regimen. The dramatic result obtained speaks for itself.

In spite of what I have just stated regarding the consumption of Pizza, I find no objection to my patients eating an *occasional* slice of pizza as long as it is prepared with natural, healthful foods such as, whole-grain flours, fresh vegetables, chicken, turkey, low fat/low salt white cheeses, mild spices and olive oil, rather than the more traditional types of ingredients, i.e. white flour, tomato sauce, sausages, salami, peppers, pepperoni, whole milk cheeses, anchovies and hot spices.

SALAD DRESSINGS—Since fresh, green, leafy vegetable salads are an important part of the diet, the types of dressings to use are a major concern to most of my patients. More than any other type, I recommend *fresh lemon juice, pure olive oil* or a *combination of the two*. Peanut, Canola, Corn, Sunflower, Sesame, Soy or Safflower Oils, in sparing amounts, may be used as an alternative to olive oil. Plain Lowfat Yogurt or Cottage Cheese, Cholesterol-Free Light Mayonnaise or commercial dressings that are 100% natural, and free of additives and preservatives may also be used. *Avoid* all dressings containing wine or grain vinegar, tomatoes or other nightshades and hot spices and seasonings. Take the time to read labels carefully. Apple cider vinegar may be added in small amounts provided that there is no adverse reaction.

Garnishes may include: finely chopped hard-boiled egg yolks, feta cheese, tofu, chopped parsley, fresh herbs, and mild spices and seasonings.

OLIVE OIL—Olive oil carries more benefits than any other oil on the market. Recent studies classify olive oil as a mono-unsaturated fatty acid that reduces levels of artery-clogging cholesterol in the blood.

Heart attacks are relatively rare in the Mediterranean countries, such as Greece and Italy. According to Dr. Scott Grundy of the University of Texas Health Science Center in Dallas, it is because olive oil is used in large quantities for cooking. This holds true for peanut oil as well.

In another article entitled, "Olive Oil May Protect The Heart,"[6] by William A. McGarey, M.D., Director of the A.R.E. Clinic in Phoenix, Arizona, the work of Dr. Grundy is discussed along with a discourse on the benefits of olive oil as perceived in the Edgar Cayce material. Dr. McGarey not only concurs that olive oil may be helpful in reducing blood fat, but also views it as a food that lubricates and nourishes the intestinal tract and is an effective blood-builder.

The Cayce material further expounds upon the benefits of olive oil for proper assimilation and elimination, acidity in the stomach and intestinal tract, colitis, and other disease entities related to the intestinal tract.

Is it any wonder that olive oil is placed high on the list of desirable foods for the psoriatic as well as the general public?

SHELLFISH (Lobster, Shrimp, Clams, Oysters, Crabs, Scallops, Snails, Mussels, etc.)—My research suggests that all psoriatic and eczema patients should totally *avoid* shellfish and sauces made with shellfish. In addition, it should be noted that Squid (Calamari), even though it does not appear to have a shell, is also classified as a shellfish. Although low in fat, Squid contains the highest amount of cholesterol to calorie ratio.

According to the June 1987 Tufts University Diet & Nutrition Letter,[7] *all* shellfish are extremely *low* in fat as well as calories, contrary to a long-time popular belief that they were high in both fat and calories. Jacob Exler, Ph.D., who wrote a handbook on shellfish for the U.S. Department of Agriculture, states that only about 0.5 to 2 percent of shellfish is fat.

In lieu of the above, we cannot attribute the adverse effects of shellfish, in the case of psoriatic and eczema cases, necessarily, to their fat content. In my opinion, it is quite significant to note that shellfish contains high quantities of *purine bodies*. The end-product of the metabolism of purine compounds is uric acid. Elevated levels of uric acid are generally associated with gout. It has been noted that in some cases of psoriasis, secondary gout may be precipitated when the uric acid in the blood is elevated (Hyperuricemia).[8] Therefore, I do not find it unreasonable to suspect the purine bodies contained in shellfish as the culprit in triggering an allergic-like reaction in psoriasis and/or eczema patients.

FISH—POULTRY (FOWL)—LAMB

Fish, Poultry and Lamb are the more readily digestible forms of animal protein and should, therefore, constitute part of the 20% acid-formers which the body needs daily.

FISH

Fish is highly recommended because it is a major source of vitamins, minerals and proteins. It is easily digestible and contains Omega-3 fatty acids which prevent cholesterol and other blood fats from building up on the walls of the arteries. Much desired fish oils are best obtained by eating fish rather than depending on fish food supplements. The best source of Omega-3 regarding seafood is fresh or canned Salmon, Sardines and Solid White Albacore. Practically all species of fish are beneficial, especially the white-fleshed, cold salt water varieties. Some fish, however, do have a high fat content, such as herring. I advise my patients to avoid such species that are known to be high in fat for reasons that do not have to be repeated.

Fish may be broiled, grilled, baked, poached, steamed—*but not fried.* A four to six ounce portion should be served at least four times a week. (A four ounce serving is approximately the size of a woman's palm.) Fresh fish is always preferred, however, frozen fish is acceptable.

SUGGESTIONS: Albacore (Solid White)—Bass—Codfish—Mahi-Mahi—Flounder—Fluke—Grouper—Haddock—Halibut—Perch—Red Snapper—Salmon—Sardines (Fresh preferred)—Scrod—Sole—Sturgeon—Swordfish—Trout—Tuna—Tilefish—Whitefish

Not Recommended: Dark-Fleshed Fish (Mackerel, Blue Fish, etc.)—Raw Fish (Sushi)—Caviar (Fish Roe)—Lox—Anchovies—Pickled or Creamed Herring—(Any Salted, Dried, Smoked or Pickled Fish)—Shellfish (Clams, Crabs, Lobster, Mussels, Oysters, Scallops, Shrimp, Squid, etc.)—Coated Fish (Breaded or Battered)—Fried or Blackened (Cajun-Style) Fish—Sauces made from Shellfish (Red or White Clam Sauce, Lobster or Shrimp Sauce, etc.)—Seasoning with hot spices, Paprika or cooking with any other nightshade.

POULTRY (FOWL)

Chicken, Turkey, Cornish Hens and other types of Non-Fatty Wild Fowl, i.e. Pheasant, Guinea Hens, Quail, etc., are also recommended. Poultry may be prepared by any low-fat cooking method, such as Broiling, Steaming, Poaching, Baking, Roasting, Grilling and Boiling—it should not be Fried. Any form of poultry may be cooked with the skin left on, however, the skin should always be removed before eating. According to Margaret Hoke, Supervisory Nutritionist at the U.S. Department of Agriculture's Human Nutrition Information Service, there is no indication that fat migrates from the skin to the meat during the cooking process.[9] Skinless white meat is preferred; the dark meat may be eaten on occasion. No more than a four to six ounce portion, per serving, approximately twice a week is suggested.

Not recommended: Fatty Fowl (Duck, Goose, etc.)—Poultry Skin—Dark Meat (in cases of Gout)—Fried or Smoked Poultry—Any Poultry that has not been thoroughly cooked—Poultry that is Battered, Breaded or Heavily Floured—Deep-Fried Poultry—Poultry that is highly seasoned or served with Cream Sauces, Gravies or Hot Spices—Garnishing or Cooking with Paprika, Tomatoes, Peppers, White Potatoes or Eggplant (NIGHTSHADES) when preparing any poultry dish.

LAMB

The only Red Meat that I suggest that my patients consume is Lamb, which is relatively easy to digest and is a high source of protein. No more than a four to six ounce serving, once or twice a week is suggested. Lamb may be cooked by Broiling, Roasting or Grilling, but again, not Fried and should be served well-done. All visible fat should be removed prior to cooking and before eating.

Not Recommended: Any other Red Meat (Beef, Pork, Veal and all products made with these meats, such as, Hamburgers, Sausage, Frankfurters, Salami, Ham, Bologna, Pastrami, Corned Beef, Kielbasa, Knockwurst, and other similarly prepared meats)—Visceral Meats (Heart, Brains, Kidney, Liver, Sweetbreads)—Combining large portions of Starches (Bread, Peas, Corn, Rice, Winter Squash, etc.) with Lamb.

Note: Even though Pork and Pork Products are not permitted, an *occasional* slice of very crisp bacon is allowed.

DAIRY PRODUCTS

Dairy Products are generally permitted provided that they are either Nonfat or Lowfat and Low in Sodium. They should always be consumed in limited and sparing amounts.

Some of my patients, particularly those that are prone to arthritis, especially psoriatic arthritis, often experience adverse reactions when consuming any type of dairy product. Symptoms, such as constipation, diarrhea, joint pains, stiffness, swelling of the hands, ankles or feet, and indigestion, indicate intolerance to this type of food. Should one or more of these reactions occur, I advise that patient to refrain from consuming dairy products altogether. Alternate sources of calcium are readily available from such foods as: Tofu, Dried Figs, Raisins, Dates, Celery, Lettuce, Turnip Greens, Kale and Sesame Seeds.

I have often observed that a patient may either develop, or already have, a preexisting intolerance to dairy foods at one point in time, but mysteriously, may not demonstrate any symptoms at another time. Therefore, the best route to take is to follow the dictates of one's own body. To reiterate—should a reaction occur, I suggest that particular patient completely eliminate consuming any dairy product; if no reaction occurs, dairy products may be included in the daily diet in limited quantities and as long as they are low in fat and salt content.

Suggestions:

Milk—Skim, Lowfat or Nonfat Milk, Buttermilk, Powdered (Dry) Milk; Goat's Milk (especially for those suffering from Eczema); Soya Milk and Almond Milk (Non-Dairy)

Eggs—Poached, Coddled, Soft or Hard-Boiled (NOT FRIED) —2 to 4 per Week

Butter—Sweet or Unsalted; Almond or Sesame Butter (Non-Dairy)

Margarine—Lowfat, Low-Salt—Made from Cold-Pressed Oils, e.g. Corn, Olive, Sesame, Safflower, Sunflower

Cheese—Lowfat, Low-Sodium White Cheese only

Cottage Cheese and Cream Cheese—Plain, Lowfat, Low-Sodium

Sour Cream and Yogurt—Plain, Non-Fat or Lowfat

Not Recommended:

• Any type of Whole Milk Dairy Product
• Dairy Products high in Fat, Sugar or Salt content; Artificial Dairy Products
• Light, Heavy, or Whipped Cream; Ice Cream and Ice Milk
• Orange and Artificially Colored Cheese
• Salted, Processed, or Imitation Butter; Hydrogenated Margarine

- Fried Eggs

- Sweetening any dairy product with Cane Sugars, Artificial Syrups or Chocolate Flavorings

- Puddings and Custards made with Whole Milk

- Combining dairy products (e.g. Milk, Cheese or Yogurt) with Citrus Fruits and their Juices, or Stewed and Dried Fruit

- Consuming any dairy product if it produces an allergic reaction

GRAINS

The advice I give my patients regarding grains is simple:

1. Avoid white bread and all other products made with white flour.

2. Whole Grain products are permitted but should not be overdone since they are all acid-formers, with the exception of Millet which is alkaline.

   Whole Grains, therefore should be part of the 20% ratio of foods permitted in the daily diet. The bran (coverings) and the germ (seed) of the grain contain the vitamins, minerals and protein. Whole grains act as a good eliminant due to their high-fiber content.

Examples of permitted grains are: Oats, Barley, Millet, Buckwheat, Rye, Groats (Kasha), Bran, Wheat (Whole, Crushed, Cracked, Bulgur, Wheat Germ), Corn and Corn Meal, Rice (Brown and Wild) and Whole Seeds (Pumpkin, Sesame, Sunflower, Flaxseed).

[Note: For best nutritional value, seeds should be soaked in water 24 hours before eating—but should be avoided altogether if a patient has an underlying diverticulosis problem.]

Products made from whole grains include: Breads, Cereals (Hot or Cold), Muffins, Bagels, Crackers, Pretzels, Pancakes and Waffles, Cookies, Cakes, Pie Crusts, Pasta, Rice and recently, even Pizza.

Suggestions:

Breads, Muffins and Bagels made of Whole Grain: Oats, Bran, Whole and Cracked Wheat, Rye, Pumpernickel, Oat Bran, etc. These products are best when toasted and, if desired, *lightly* spread with Unsalted (Sweet) Butter, Lowfat Margarine (made from Cold-Pressed Oils), Lowfat Cream Cheese and/or a little Honey or Natural Fruit Preserves.

Cereals (High-Fiber/Whole Grain) such as: Bran, Whole Wheat (Cracked, Crushed), Millet, Oat Bran, Oats (Rolled, Cracked and Steel Cut), Bulgur Wheat, etc.

Hot or Cold Cereals: Examples—Cream of Wheat, Shredded Wheat, Puffed Wheat, Ralston, Oatmeal, Maltex, Wheatena, Nutri-Grain, Seven-Grain Cereal, Uncle Sam Cereal, Total, etc.

[Note: Hot Cereals should not be over cooked as this will destroy the vitamin/mineral content.]

Additives may include:

Skim or Lowfat Milk, Wheat Germ, Cinnamon, Slivered or Chopped Almonds, a little Honey, Pure Maple Syrup or Molasses (both sparingly). Also any fruit (other than Raw Apples, Bananas, Melon, Citrus, Dried or Stewed Fruit) may be added, but in limited amounts. Strawberries are not permitted in cases of Psoriatic Arthritis.

Perhaps the most important basic rules to remember are:

1.   Do not combine Citrus Fruits or Citrus Juices at the same meal with Whole Grains, and

2.   Avoid any Whole Grain product if it creates an allergic reaction.

Pasta is a favorite in practically every country on earth. There is no reason why the psoriatic cannot enjoy pasta dishes provided the pasta is whole-grain or vegetable in its makeup (no white flour pasta).

Most recommended pastas are: American (Jerusalem) Artichoke, Carrot, Spinach, Corn, Soya Egg, Mung Bean, Whole Wheat and Buckwheat Noodles. Cellophane Rice Noodles are good substitute for regular white flour Spaghetti, Macaroni and Noodles. Newer products, such as, Saffron

Noodles and Parsley/Garlic Pasta are constantly finding their way onto the shelves of supermarkets as well as specialty gourmet shops.

They may be prepared with Mild Herbs and Spices—Fresh, Steamed or Cooked Vegetables (Pasta Primavera)—Pesto Sauce (Basil, Garlic, Olive Oil, Almonds or Pine Nuts)—or an Olive Oil/Garlic Sauce.

Always AVOID sauces made from: Tomatoes, Butter, Cream, Shellfish (White or Red), and Hot Spices.

Pizza—Another favorite, particularly in America, is permitted on occasion only if it is made from natural products and not the traditional ingredients. As discussed earlier, the most popular type of pizza contain practically every product that plays havoc with a person suffering from psoriasis; namely, Tomatoes, White Flour, Peppers, Processed Meat, Whole Milk Cheese, etc.

The type I permit my patients to indulge in once in a while strangely enough is gaining popularity and is referred to as "Health-Food Pizza." The ingredients include Whole-Grain Pie Crust, Lowfat Cheese, and toppings with Fresh Vegetables and at times Chicken and Turkey chunks. Once again, I stress to my patients that even though this item contains "permitted" foods they should still not go overboard. Remember—all things in moderation.

Rice is a world staple. It is found throughout all corners of the earth. Its value in sustaining the human race, particularly in the Far East, is without equal.

There really is only one thing to remember about rice in cases of psoriasis and that is to avoid eating white rice. Instead of white, polished rice, I advise my patients to consume only Brown or Wild Rice. It must be remembered however that rice, being a grain is acid-forming—so—once again, enjoy it—but not to excess. It may be cooked by boiling or steaming but not fried.

Whole-Grain Rice Cakes make a good snack. Examples are: Rye, Sesame, Buckwheat, Multi-Grain, etc.—again, white rice cakes are to be avoided.

Toppings on Rice Cakes could include: Honey (1 tsp.), Natural Fruit Jams, Jellies, and Preserves (1 tsp.), Lowfat White Cheese (1 slice), Lowfat Ricotta or Cottage Cheese (1 tsp.), White Meat Turkey or Chicken (1 slice), Plain Lowfat Yogurt, or any Non-Citrus Fruit.

Crackers, Pretzels and Popcorn are often asked about by my patients. I suggest to them the following: Unsalted Matzos, Rye Crisp, Lowfat/Unsalted Saltines, Unsalted Wheat and Oat Bran Crackers, Unsalted Whole-Grain Pretzels and Unsalted, Unbuttered Air-Popped Popcorn.

In general, therefore, the basic thing to remember about grains is to enjoy them in moderation, choose only the whole-grain products, avoid the white flour products and do not mix cereals and citrus products at the same meal. If one abides by these simple rules, grains will not be a problem, in fact, they will add to the enjoyment and nutritional value of the daily diet.

SWEETS

FOR THE SWEET TOOTH—It is of the utmost importance that psoriatic, psoriatic arthritic, and eczema sufferers eliminate most fats as well as sugary sweets and white flour products (sugary cereals, frostings, candy, regular or diet sodas, etc.) from their diet. There are, however, natural and nutritious substitutes that will satisfy the body's craving for sweets, such as:

Fresh fruit or fruit salads—Dried, unsulphured tropical fruits—Stewed or cooked fruits (figs, prunes, apricots, apples, etc.)—Homemade apple sauce or 100% natural store-bought apple sauce—Baked apple sweetened with honey, maple syrup, or a sprinkling of brown sugar and cinnamon—Fruit juices (grape, pear, apricot and papaya)—Knox Unflavored Gelatin combined with diced fruit, water and fruit juice—Plain low fat yogurt with fruit, low fat frozen yogurt—Fresh fruit sorbets—100% natural frozen fruit bars—All Natural, whole-grain cookies.

Honey, one of nature's most perfect foods, as well as pure maple syrup and molasses is permitted if consumed in small amounts. These sweeteners serve as an excellent topping for breads, muffins and cereals.

NOTE: CAROB, contrary to popular belief, *is not* a good substitute for chocolate. According to the Center for Science in the Public Interest, carob is saturated with fat and may be even more conducive to heart disease than beef fat.

Since sweets are generally acid-formers, they should be selected carefully. The *natural* sweets derived mainly from fresh or dried fruits can supply the sugars necessary to form the alcohol needed for proper digestion and assimilation.

If, for any reason, the suggestions above do not fulfill my patients' craving for sweets, I allow them the flexibility of indulging themselves, once in a while, by having a *small* portion of their favorite dessert.

Artificial Sweeteners—For several years, specific artificial sweeteners, such as saccharin, have been brought under the scrutiny of the F.D.A. as possible cancer producers. The November 1985 edition of The Journal of the American Medical Association, however, presented findings regarding this subject matter. The article clearly vindicated saccharin as a cancer producer and stated that the evidence does not support a link to cancer in humans. The report by the A.M.A's Council on Scientific Matters further declared that: "Available evidence indicates that ... saccharin is not associated with an increased risk of bladder cancer." It further stated that "The A.M.A. is not implying that it condones the use of saccharin." It did, however, support the sweetener's availability as a food additive.

Earlier, in July 1985, the A.M.A. concluded that the normal use of another artificial sweetener, aspartame, sold on the market as Nutra-Sweet, was not associated with serious health problems. Reports have been filtering down, however, on the adverse effects that Nutra-Sweet has had on some individuals in the form of headache, dizziness and seizures, especially in teenagers. Only time and further research will settle this issue.

In general, therefore, I do permit my patients to use artificial sweeteners, but only in minimal amounts. I always remind them that the ultimate effect artificial products have on the human body is still a controversial subject.

BEVERAGES

Liquid intake, especially pure water, should be of primary interest to the psoriatic. The bathing of the cells, the flushing of the kidneys, the movements throughout the small and large intestines, and the chemical processes of the body are to a great extent, if not completely, dependent upon a healthy, fluid environment. It goes without saying that the type of liquid intake chosen should be relatively free of toxins, pollutants, destructive artificial additives, preservatives, colorings, or any other potentially harmful product. The optimum is to select those liquids that are cleansing and healthful which enhance, rather than hinder, these vital body processes.

Water—During the preliminary consultation with so many of my new psoriasis patients, I am nothing less than amazed to find that they rarely, if ever, drink pure water daily. In fact, it is unusual to even meet someone who drinks more than one or two glasses a day. Most people feel that their daily water intake is adequately supplied through the foods they eat or by other liquids, such as diet soda, alcohol, beer, coffee, tea, etc. Obviously, there are many individuals, without chronic skin conditions, whose bodies can apparently handle such an accumulation of toxins. In cases of psoriasis or eczema, however, such a violation can only aggravate an already over-polluted system.

I am not one to harp on "rules" but if ever there was a so-called rule that I insist be followed, especially for a psoriatic, it is: *Drink 6 to 8 eight-ounce glasses of pure water a day, in addition to all other beverages consumed.*

Water is not only convenient, inexpensive and calorie-free, but also can effectively curb one's appetite. Whenever hungry, or before a meal, I suggest drinking a glass of water first. Because it is tasteless, water can also help break the desire for sweet-tasting foods and beverages.

As an alternative to just plain water, I recommend that my patients add the juices of 4 or 5 fresh lemons or limes to a gallon of spring, filtered or bottled water. It should then be refrigerated and consumed whenever desired. This will help the body processes in cleansing, lubrication and alkalinity. [Refer to "The Importance of Water" in Chapter, INTERNAL CLEANSING.]

FRUIT AND VEGETABLE JUICES—Unsweetened fruit juices and vegetable juices are to be consumed as often as possible. If a rash occurs or the skin becomes sensitive due to drinking too much orange or grapefruit juice (citrus), drink less or eliminate them.

All juices should either be freshly made or, if store-bought, purchased in a glass container or wax carton. Avoid any *canned juices.*

A few drops to a quarter of a cup of lemon or lime juice should be added to a 6—8 oz. glass of orange juice or grapefruit juice. Pure grape juice, as well as other nutritious juices such as, pineapple, pear, papaya, mango and apricot are also recommended. Combinations of these juices are also suggested.

Vegetable juices as well as fruit juices are best freshly made in a home juicer. There is one major restriction regarding vegetable juices: *Avoid tomato juice and all juices that contain tomato.*

Occasionally adding one (1) packet of Knox Unflavored Gelatin to a glass of fruit or vegetable juice will help to insure maximum nutritional absorption.

Always keep in mind that consuming too much of any one food item, even if it is on the permitted list, can produce a toxicity in the body. For instance, too many carrots or drinking too much carrot juice can produce Hypercarotenemia bringing about pseudo-jaundice. An overabundance of fruit can raise the tri-glyceride level of the blood which can cause a skin reaction. In other words, avoid extremes!

COFFEE—The debate on the effects coffee has on the human organism has been going on for 30 years. Finally, in 1986, scientific data was released to the public which indicated that anyone who consumed more than 3 cups of coffee per day was at risk of impairing calcium absorption as well as developing heart disease. According to another study by the Johns Hopkins Medical School in Baltimore, anyone who drinks 5 or more cups of coffee a day has more than twice the risk of having heart problems than someone who drinks no coffee at all. This survey was conducted on 1,000 men over a twenty-five year period.

In October of 1990, however, new findings published in the New England Journal of Medicine, completely refutes the previous findings when a study of more than 45,000 men found no evidence that coffee boosts the risk of heart disease or stroke.

What is one to do? Follow the experts and you find yourself in a state of confusion. Do whatever you please and you may jeopardize your health.

Consequently, I feel that using plain common sense is the answer. I suggest that for those of my patients who feel a need to drink coffee, that they consume no more than 3 cups of black, decaffeinated coffee per day, without milk, cream or sugar. For those that have little or no desire for coffee, I recommend eliminating it from one's diet altogether—period!

It seems to me that the question here is not whether coffee in itself is harmful, but rather how much is consumed. An unreasonable amount can lead not only to physical, but mental reactions as well.

Case in Point

Mr. A.G. came into my office on September 18, 1985, suffering from a rather severe degree of psoriasis which he had had for twenty years. The primary areas involved were across the upper area of his back, shoulders, and down each arm. What disturbed him most, however, was the severity of the disease throughout his hands. His profession involved being in close contact with the general public. Because of his embarrassment, he would take whatever measures that were necessary to avoid exposing his hands.

Rarely, have I had such a cooperative patient. Without question or complaint, he did everything that was required. Although the progress was slow, it was steady. In a few months, his back, shoulders and most of his upper arms cleared up nicely—however, the tops of his hands showed no change. He noticed that during the week, the lesions of his hands would not be so inflamed; on weekends, however, they would flare up to an intolerable degree. This pattern repeated itself every week.

We sat down and tried to figure out the reason for this recurrence. Was there something that A.G. was doing, or perhaps not doing, that caused this adverse reaction to occur only on weekends? There was—he drank too much coffee.

It seems that during the week when he was busy working as a traveling salesman, he would drink seven to ten cups of coffee a day. On weekends, when he was an auctioneer, which placed him under a great deal of tension, he admitted to drinking as much as sixteen or seventeen cups a day! There was no need to look any further. I reminded him that although black coffee was permitted on the diet, drinking sixteen cups a day was utterly ridiculous. The maximum that I allowed was three cups per day. Mr. A.G. decided not only to cut down on his coffee intake on weekends but to refrain from drinking it altogether. He proved to me that when he made up his mind to do something, he did it.

Results were not immediate. Three weeks passed without any apparent change in his condition. I was ready to give up the idea that coffee was the culprit when a change began to take place. The remaining lesions on the lower arms began drying up. He began to feel better in general, with his energy level greatly improving. Most important of all, were the changes that occurred in his hands. The irritation on the tops of his hands was hardly visible. I, as well as he, was now convinced that the excessive amounts of coffee that he drank on weekends was the primary reason for the flare-ups.

This, however, is not the end of the story; there was a fringe benefit. Not only did his hands clear up, but so did his disposition. On July 21, 1986, his wife accompanied him to my office and expounded on how pleasant he had become compared to a few weeks earlier. He concurred with her, and in addition, recognized that he was now able to handle his business affairs in a much more relaxed manner. What had previously disturbed him and seemed almost insurmountable was now taken in stride and handled with much more ease. One can only conclude that because of the high concentration of caffeine in his system, he was always in an uptight mental, as well as physical state. Once the caffeine was no longer ingested, his thinking became clearer and his everyday challenges were met with greater confidence.

AUTHOR'S NOTE: Although 3 cups of coffee are allowed on the diet per day, I have personally notated that by eliminating coffee altogether, several of my patients reported a marked beneficial reaction to their skin. As a substitute for coffee, some patients drank a cup of hot water with the juice of a lemon or lime which seemed to satisfy them.

HERB TEAS—The teas involved in helping to heal psoriasis and eczema are natural herb teas which affect the internal cleansing process and aid in the restoration of the intestinal walls. Most herbal teas do not contain caffeine, theobromide, or tannin, all potentially harmful ingredients that can lead to nervousness, insomnia, rapid heartbeat, and disruption of blood sugar levels. Popular commercial teas, however, do contain these unhealthy elements and should therefore be avoided.

The most beneficial herb teas suggested are:

1. American Yellow (not Spanish) Saffron Tea

2. Slippery Elm Bark Powder

Substitutes for American Yellow Saffron Tea are:

Camomile Tea

Mullein Tea

Watermelon Seed Tea

[Details regarding these teas and their preparation appear in the next chapter, "Herb Teas."]

MILK—Generally, milk is hard to digest and can be constipating. It produces a great deal of mucus. In the training of athletes where good respiration is essential, whole milk is usually eliminated from their diets. Milk is not considered to be an acid-former, therefore, it is included in the diet but only in the form of Skim or Lowfat Milk and milk in its predigested form such as Lowfat Buttermilk and Lowfat Yogurt. Soya or Goat's Milk has been found to be more tolerable in cases of Eczema.

CARBONATED DRINKS—Carbonated soft drinks, sodas in particular, are saturated with sugars, preservatives, artificial flavorings, and colorings. In spite of the fact that Regular and Diet Sodas contain these known detrimental ingredients, they are the most popular beverages consumed by the general public. Obviously, since purification of the blood is the keynote in the healing of psoriasis, these drinks should be viewed as poison to all psoriatics. As previously discussed in an earlier chapter, the liver is perhaps the most active filtering gland of the body. It must be in peak condition, without blockages or hindrances of any kind, in order to function properly. The excessive consumption of sodas has such a destructive effect on the liver that some authorities feel that even one glass a day is too much.

During a speaking engagement at the University of Massachusetts, Dr. S.H. Hutner stated that "cirrhosis (disease) of the liver may as often affect soft drink addicts as alcoholics." He theorizes that the "empty calories" in sugary sodas make people cut down on their consumption of wholesome foods which produces a protein deficiency resulting in cirrhosis of the liver. The standard treatment for this condition is to place the patient on a high protein, low-carbohydrate diet with vitamin supplements and eliminate all soft drinks.

As a substitute for soft drinks, I recommend drinking an occasional cold glass of *naturally carbonated water* such as Perrier or Saratoga

Water, or just plain Seltzer Water (not Club Soda). Fresh lemon or lime juice may be added to these beverages and served over ice. Not only is this cleansing to the system, but also thirst-quenching, delicious and satisfying. Many of my patients have even found this to be the solution to social drinking.

ALCOHOLIC BEVERAGES—Of all the sacrifices that a psoriatic must make, eliminating alcohol is the most difficult one, especially if the patient is a "drinker." If I find early on in my course of treatment that a patient is unwilling to accept the fact that he or she must avoid hard liquor in any form, I have no qualms in advising against further treatment.

Some years ago, a physician referred a psoriatic patient to me. She was most receptive to my suggestions and apparently followed through on all that was required of her. After only a few weeks, her psoriasis cleared up considerably, however, I never saw her again. Months went by before I met with the doctor who originally referred her to me. I informed him of her negligence in continued treatments. He nodded his head in an understanding manner and said, "John, you didn't fail, she was responding beautifully—but she simply could not give up her dry martini's. She was just too embarrassed to tell you."

In cases of psoriasis and eczema, therefore, it is extremely important that alcohol, in all its forms, including beer, be totally eliminated. The only leeway that I allow my patients regarding alcohol is drinking an occasional glass of dry red or white wine. No more than 2 to 4 oz. is permitted with dinner or with a slice of dark bread late in the afternoon. The combination of wine, especially red wine, and brown bread is a powerful blood builder according to the Cayce works. Taken in this manner, they are considered a "food." Wine, in itself, contains iron and plasm which can benefit the system. For those who prefer white wine, I suggest to them a "Spritzer" (half white wine and half seltzer with a slice of lemon over ice). Again, this is permitted only on occasion and should not become too much of a habit.

CAUTION: If a patient is on any kind of medication or suffers from Gout, wine is not permitted under any circumstances.

"Doctor, Can I Cheat?"

A question that often arises is whether or not a patient can "cheat" on the diet. The answer is that some can get away with it, while others cannot. For most patients, it is ill-advised to break the diet during the first few months of the prescribed regimen. I encourage my patents to remain on the diet until they are clear of all lesions. After this has been accomplished, they can slowly add certain types of foods to their diet that they once enjoyed. If an unfavorable reaction begins to occur, that is, a recurrence of skin eruptions, they are to immediately revert back to the recommended diet for a longer period of time. The deciding factor is whether or not the body is now capable of filtering out and removing toxins formed by acid foods.

Expect a Weight Loss

The dietary suggestions contained herein offers an added benefit that is generally welcomed by most patients—a *healthy* weight loss. Many psoriatics carry ten, twenty, thirty, or more pounds of excess baggage around with them in the form of accumulated fat. When they hear that they can and will lose weight on this diet they are more encouraged by knowing that they have an excellent opportunity of not only ridding themselves of psoriasis but also of their unwanted poundage.

Loss of excess weight has become such a consistent finding that when no weight loss is evident, it is a strong indication to me that the patient is not adequately adhering to the diet—even though they often try to deny it.

With some patients, they become alarmed when friends or relatives become over-concerned about their obvious weight loss. Usually, these well-meaning friends are simply unaccustomed to seeing a "svelte" figure appear before them. More often than not, a patient feels better than ever, has an abundance of vitality, and is able to fit into stylish clothes which, in itself, enhances their self-esteem.

For those who feel there is too much of a weight loss, I advise them to simply eat more of the "permitted" foods listed in the "80%" category, i.e. fruits, vegetables and their juices—however, *without over-indulging themselves*. It should be noted that even though it is important to be conscious of the types of foods consumed, equal emphasis should be placed on the quantity and the size of the portions eaten, as well as the proper combination of foods. All of these factors determine the effect that foods have on the system. Patients should never feel hungry by following the diet. If they do, it is simply because they are not consuming enough of the body-building foods.

Being Flexible

As important as it is to adhere to the diet *as closely as possible*, it should be maintained with a certain amount of flexibility. The entire dietary concept should not become an irritable, restrictive chore because of being overly-precise regarding every food item listed. Allowing for that expected number of failures, if my patients primarily adhere to the basic dietary suggestions long enough, they are usually successful.

Although there are certain restrictions such as, fatty foods and the nightshades, most of the diet can be followed and adhered to with a certain amount of leeway and flexibility without affecting the total, overall effect. I see no harm in allowing a patient to occasionally satisfy a desire for a specific food after being on the diet for a few weeks, as long as it is not overdone and there is no adverse reaction.

The feelings of restriction will be less intense and not as frustrating if one is determined to make the diet interesting, tasteful and as creative as possible. Presently, there are many nutritious cookbooks on the market today that contain helpful suggestions and recipes that utilize the allowed foods. Once familiar with these preparations, the entire procedure will become simpler, appealing, and consequently, more enjoyable.

Over-Eating

In order to obtain successful results with the regimen, it is important to consume only moderate-sized portions of the foods permitted. There have been some cases where over-indulging these foods has proven to be the reason for a delayed, beneficial reaction.

It is not uncommon to find that some patients who fail to respond, do so because they consume *too much* of the foods recommended, especially where meats and sweets are concerned. Consequently, as mentioned previously, there should always be a conscious awareness of the *quantity* of food intake. Simply because a food item is listed as "permitted" does not grant a patient license to "pig out."

I recall one patient, who was advised to eat *a few* almonds a day, proceeded to consume a *full pound* of nuts in one evening! His reasoning was that because they appeared on the recommended list of foods, the more he ate, the better! With still another patient who did not respond after maintaining the diet for several months, just cutting back on the *quantity* of allowed foods caused not only a desirable weight loss but cleared up all her psoriatic lesions at the same time. As the fat diminished, a sense of well-being took place, apparently because of the relief it brought to her heart, lungs, liver and skin. Therefore, when there is a choice of eating more or less—always eat less!

To my knowledge, our third President of the United States, Thomas Jefferson, did not have psoriasis, nor was he a dietician—he was a Statesman. Nevertheless, his genius should be appreciated by all in his simple statement, "We never repent of having eaten too little."

Food Allergies

Even though specific foods appear in the diet, some may not always have an agreeable effect on the patient. With some individuals, there are permitted foods that may possibly cause an allergic reaction. The Apple Diet, if you remember from my chapter "Internal Cleansing," is one of the most effective ways to cleanse the body of internal toxins. The vast majority of my patients have had no difficulty maintaining this diet for three days. However, one of my patients did advise me that eating any kind of apple could cause such a violent reaction in the form of throat constriction, that it might possibly endanger her life. Even having an apple touch her lips resulted in swelling so severe that she could barely open her mouth. Obviously, the Apple Diet was not for her. In another instance, a patient was able to eat all the carrots she wanted but could not touch them because her fingers would blister and break out in a rash. Comparable reactions have been known to occur in some patients by eating Dairy Products, Citrus Fruits and Juices, and products made of Wheat.

Therefore—*PATIENTS SHOULD AVOID ALL FOODS THAT THEY KNOW WILL HAVE A DETRIMENTAL EFFECT ON THEM EVEN THOUGH THEY ARE NOTED AS PERMITTED ON THE DIETARY LIST CONTAINED HEREIN.*

Food allergies are more common and far-reaching than ordinarily believed. Identifying personal food allergies does not fall within the scope of this book. For those interested, there are two Allergy/Sensitivity Tests available. (1) Cytotoxic Test (capable of identifying up to 250 foods or additives). (2) Leucocyte Antigen Sensitivity Test [LAST] (considered by many to be more thorough and accurate than the Cytotoxic Test). These tests should be performed only under qualified medical supervision.

Vitamin and Mineral Supplements

The question of whether or not vitamin supplements are necessary in the management of psoriasis is often asked by patients and physicians alike. My research suggests that they play only a minor role, provided that a patient adheres to all the dietary suggestions and regimen. Obtaining necessary vitamins and minerals in their natural state, i.e. foods such as, fruits and vegetables and their juices, far surpasses those obtained from natural or synthetic manufactured sources. Nevertheless, there are instances when they may be of some value, if only from a psychological point of view.

The vitamins and minerals most frequently associated with psoriasis are vitamins A with D, as well as the B vitamins. According to Melvyn R. Werbach, M.D. in his classic account, *Nutritional Influences On Illness*, during a ten year experimental psoriasis study, 118 out of 155 patients responded with purified granulated soya phosphatides. Crude lecithin, 3-6 gm. daily, was also given, in addition to small amounts of vitamins A, D, B-1, B-2, B-6, and calcium pantoghenate. When using vitamin D-3 with a control base, applied topically, 5 out of 5 patients showed "remarkable improvement." Other sources indicate that similar results have been obtained by using vitamin E topically. I found it particularly noteworthy that Dr. Werbach also cited in another experimental study that 6 out of 6 patients improved on *elimination diets*.[10]

The bottom line is that vitamin supplements may prove beneficial in some cases and generally pose no threat to the patient. Be that as it may, the patient should, however, first consult with a licensed health practitioner before embarking on a therapeutic regimen of vitamins, whether they be administered systemically or topically.

Out of Sight—Out of Mind

One of the most effective measures that one can take in making the diet easier to follow is to simply buy only those foods that are recommended and avoid purchasing the those that are not. The refrigerator and kitchen cabinets should be well stocked with these foods at all times. Obviously, if one lives alone, this is easier to do, but families, spouses and roommates who have followed this diet along with the patient have often commented to me that it was beneficial to them as well. They not only felt better generally and lost excess weight, but they were helping their friend or loved one at the same time, by encouraging him or her to maintain the diet.

When Dining Out

Unquestionably, there are many people who, because of their professions, occupations or life-styles, eat many or most of their meals in restaurants. Even so, it is not impossible to have your food specially prepared when eating out is a necessity. Currently, there are many restaurants that are conscious of individual preferences and will gladly accommodate their patrons by preparing foods according to their wishes. I encourage my patients to take advantage of this and make their desires known.

I suggest the following to my patients when dining out:

- Select foods that are Steamed, Broiled, Stir-Fried, Poached, Baked, Grilled or Cooked in their own juices.

- Avoid ordering Fried, Blackened, Buttered, Creamed, "Au Gratin," Breaded foods and those with rich sauces.

- Ask the waiter how a dish is prepared.

- Request that the Chef avoid buttering before broiling, to serve salad dressings on the side and to substitute lowfat for high-fat cheese.

- Trim off all visible fat on meats and poultry before eating. Remove skin from poultry before eating; it may however be cooked with the skin on.

- Order Fish, Non-Fatty Fowl or Lamb. Do not order Beef, Pork, Veal or Shellfish.

- Select whole-grain breads, bread sticks and bagels rather than the high-fat croissants, cornbread or biscuits.

- Order "a la carte" whenever possible so that you may be more selective.

- To satisfy a sweet tooth, order fresh fruit, lowfat frozen yogurt, naturally-sweetened fruit ices, or any other type of lowfat dessert.

- When dining in Italian Restaurants, order menu items described as "affogato" (steamed or poached).

- In Chinese Restaurants, order steamed vegetable dishes, poached fish dishes and steamed poultry dishes. Avoid eating beef, pork or shellfish dishes and foods prepared with MSG (monosodium glutamate).

- Avoid ordering hot, spicy dishes. Select the more simply prepared entrees.

- Always order a large green leafy salad, such as a garden salad, but avoid eating the nightshades. Salad dressing most preferred is olive oil and lemon juice.

Out of the Past

It is not that effective results in psoriasis with dietary changes have never been reported by serious researchers or observers in the past, but rather it is that their reports have been largely overlooked, minimized, or simply ignored.

Consider the following:

1. Dr. L. Duncan Bulkley, M.D., in his speech to the Section of Dermatology of the A.M.A. in the early 1900's stated that the proper diet for the treatment of psoriasis is low protein, vegetarian. He believed that there had to be a cause for these diseases which, once found and eliminated, would lead to a disappearance of the disease. Diet, he felt, often played a key role.

2. Dr. Hans J. Schwartz, M.D. in 1926 reports in the *Archives of Dermatology* (p. 672-4), "Association of Intestinal Indigestion with Various Dermatoses" concludes that, after studying 900 cases suffering from skin problems, an important causative factor was excess toxins in the system. These patients were consuming foods primarily protein or carbohydrates, in excess of their body's needs.

3. In 1927, Dr. J. Frederick Burgess, M.D., a lecturer in Dermatology at McGill University and Associate Dermatologist of Montreal General Hospital, confirmed the findings of Dr. Schwartz. He concluded: "While eczema may result from 'external irritant' causes, internal irritants which may be formed in the intestines as a result of bacterial decomposition are also capable of acting as skin irritants..."

4. Dr. James Galloway, M.D., writing in the British Medical Journal as early as 1913 (p. 815-817) observed the same phenomenon.

5. In a 1932 volume of the *Journal of the American Medical Association* (JAMA), Dr. Jay F. Schamberg, M.D., then a Professor of Dermatology at the Graduate School of Medicine at the University of Pennsylvania, described how he had treated psoriasis: "a low protein diet, without any other internal or external treatment, causes a disappearance of the greater part of the eruptions..." This respected physician, along with others, worked extensively with many patients who suffered from psoriasis. Photographs taken before and after a change in his patient's diets accompany his article. "These photographs," notes Dr. Schamberg, "constitute to my mind irrefutable documentary evidence of the truth of the statement that a low protein diet has an enormous influence on the course of the psoriatic eruption."

It follows that the next most logical questions is—if they knew this as far back as the turn of the century, why are so many psoriasis patients still suffering with the disease. My answer to that is that their research, for one reason or another, stopped there. They simply did not go far enough. They observed that diet played a decided role in the alleviation of psoriasis, but they could not reason why. Consequently, they were unable to attack the root cause of the disease. Cayce was able to take us "One Step Beyond" and not only pinpoint the cause as a thinning of the intestinal walls, but advise on what to do about it—the major remedy being proper diet, nutrition and internal cleansing.

Nevertheless, the answer evades me as to why this avenue was not pursued relentlessly at that time since they had impressive evidence that indicated diet played a significant role in controlling psoriasis. After all, it was the same disease then as it is today, albeit, the toxins may differ somewhat. To this day, if a dermatologist, especially a researcher, is asked about diet relative to psoriasis, their worn-out answer in practically every instance is, "There is no scientific evidence that diet plays a significant role in the healing of psoriasis, etc., etc., etc.," to which I answer, "Oh! But there is. Turn back the pages and examine the research conducted by your own colleagues and you will find there is indeed a diet/psoriasis relationship." Admittedly, the answer is not always as simple as applying a cream, light-box or drug, but the results are overwhelmingly in favor of this natural alternative.

I fully concur, mind you, that it is hard to believe that a devastating illness, such as severe psoriasis, can be completely alleviated by something as simple as a change of diet—especially since such sophisticated present day therapies are available. Actually, it doesn't matter if you want to believe it or not; the truth is the truth. In the majority of patients I have cared for, that *is* the case. Rather than criticize the concept, the psoriasis patients I have encountered looked upon the idea as a godsend, a way out of their dilemma, especially when such a revelation is backed up by irrefutable evidence.

To summarize, since the turn of the century, perhaps even sooner, undeniable results have been attained in cases of psoriasis by observing some basic rules of nutrition: A low protein, vegetarian diet, no refined foods, high in raw fruits and vegetables, lowfat, high fiber foods.

Cayce's concepts to counteract skin problems ran astonishingly close to those of the experts (at least in days gone by). He declared in #563-4, *"...do not use fats or highly seasoned foods but [rather] those that tend to be more of an alkaline nature..."* He also advised having very little sweets—to avoid cane sugar altogether. Drink 6 to 8 glasses of pure water daily as well as eating *2 to 4 raw almonds a day* and you have much of the Cayce basic formula from a dietary point of view, for correcting or avoiding most skin problems.

In view of the above, one can only conclude that *dietary violations are the primary causative factors in skin diseases.*

Author's Comments

Common sense must always be exercised when following any nutritional regimen. To reiterate, if a particular food does not agree with any of my patients, even if it appears on the "permitted" food list, it is avoided. If feelings of weakness or hunger are present, they simply eat more of the body-building foods but *never* to the point of being gluttonous. In short, discipline should be maintained in the *quantity* as well as the *quality* (type) of food consumed.

As an effective support system, I usually suggest that my patients, while in the early stages of the regimen, interact with other psoriatics who have been pleased with their results. This networking has proven to be perhaps the most positive and encouraging influence in convincing new patients that proper nutrition is a major tool in controlling the disease.

It has become obvious by now that select foods play a most significant role in healing psoriasis. The scientific community must eventually acknowledge the role that nutrition plays in skin diseases.

Psoriatics, the world over, should take heed to the wisdom of Hippocrates, The Father of Medicine:

"LET YOUR FOOD BE YOUR MEDICINE—
LET YOUR MEDICINE BE YOUR FOOD."

FURTHER NUTRITIONAL ADVICE I OFFER MY PATIENTS
CAN BE FOUND IN APPENDIX A

REFERENCES
(Chapter 6—Diet and Nutrition)

1. Edgar Cayce Reference # 306-3, (Virginia Beach, VA, The Edgar Cayce Foundation, copyright 1971) Reprinted by permission.
2. Israel S. Kleiner, Ph.D., *Human Biochemistry*, (St. Louis, The C.V. Mosby Co., copyright 1954, ed. 4) pg. 543.
3. Francis Marion Pottenger, M.D., *Symptoms of Visceral Disease*, (St. Louis, The C.V. Mosby Co., 1953, ed. 7) p. 144. Reprinted by permission.
4. Adelle Davis, *Let's Get Well*, (New York, NY, Harcourt, Brace & World, Inc. 1965) p. 156.
5. Michael Gauguelin, *How Atmospheric Conditions Affect Your Health*, (New York, NY, Stein and Day Publishers, 7 East 48th Street).
6. William A. McGarey, M.D., "Olive Oil May Protect The Heart," *Pathways to Health* (Phoenix, AZ, The A.R.E. Clinic, Inc., Vol. 7, No. 3) By permission.
7. "Shucking the Myth About Cholesterol in Shellfish"—*Tufts University Diet and Nutrition Letter* (Food for Thought—Vol. 5—No. 4, June 1987) p. 7. By permission.
8. Eugene J. Van Scott, M.D. and Eugene M. Farber, M.D., *Dermatology in General Medicine* (New York, NY, 1971, McGraw-Hill Inc.) Chapter 8—p. 226.
9. "More than one way to skin a chicken"—*Tufts University Diet and Nutrition Letter* (Food for Thought—Vol. 8—No. 10, December 1990) p. 7.
10. Melvyn R. Werbach, M.D., *Nutritional Influence on Illness*, (New Canaan, CN, Keats Publishing, Inc., copyright 1987-1988) pg. 372.

Chapter 7

Herb Teas

As a boy I was fascinated by the adventures of Tarzan in the famous stories by Edgar Rice Burroughs. I was particularly in awe of Tarzan's ability to heal the injured and ill with herbal medicines. For reasons I could not explain, the way Tarzan was able to cure both internal and external ailments by extracting juices from various herbs, and then either applying them directly to a wound, or administering them orally, seemed to ring true.

The Tarzan stories were fiction, of course, but were this primitive jungle physician's methods so farfetched? When one stops to think about it, all we have in this plane of existence, from a physical point of view, is derived from the earth. Herbs and herb teas have been used for healing since the dawn of human history, and most of our modern drugs are still derived from plants. Our medicines today typically come in capsule form, carefully measured and attractively packaged, but they still have their origins in Nature.

Herbal healing is the oldest form of healing on earth. Throughout the Bible, passages advocating the use of herbs as part of the daily diet are numerous. Some writers say there is an herb for every disease that afflicts mankind. Hippocrates (born 460 B.C.) proved that many diseases can be treated successfully by natural means alone. According to historical data, herbs, diet, and baths were the mainstay of his treatments.

The North American Indians, as well as peoples of other ancient cultures, have also made extensive use of herbs to cure many diseases and still do. Presently there is a growing appreciation for the medicinal value of herbs in their natural form, and their use in both poultices and herbal drinks is again gaining wide acceptance. In this chapter we are particularly concerned with the herbs suggested for psoriasis sufferers in the form of tea.

Commercial teas as we know them today contain caffeine, theobromide, and tannin all potentially harmful to the body. As stated earlier, they can lead to nervousness, insomnia, rapid heart beat, and disruption of blood sugar levels if very potent and used in large quantities. In contrast, most herb teas do not contain these potentially harmful ingredients, and some of them are very helpful in clearing psoriasis. Five specific herbs are recommended for this purpose. Named in order of their importance they are: (1) Saffron (American Yellow), (2) Ground slippery elm bark, (3) Camomile, (4) Mullein, and (5) Watermelon Seed Tea.

Saffron Tea (carthamus tinctorius):

The saffron called for in cases of psoriasis is the *American yellow*, not the "true" or Spanish saffron (crocus sativus), which is grown not only in Spain but also in western Asia, France, and Austria. Most patients would probably be shocked at the cost of Spanish saffron which sells for approximately $25 an ounce. This is because it takes about 75,000 flowers to make one pound. Its value was known even in the time of Solomon three thousand years ago when it was used as a dye, in scented salves, and as an aromatic placed in the Greek halls and courts, and in the Roman baths. Today, because of its expense, it is seldom used except for certain medicinal purposes and (primarily) as a flavoring in certain dishes.

American yellow saffron, often substituted for the Spanish variety, is produced mostly in America, England, and the countries surrounding the Mediterranean Sea. For the psoriatic it is better than the Spanish, modest in price (only five dollars for two ounces) and is easier to find, a welcomed fact for all patients.

Saffron tea is the kind most frequently prescribed for a variety of ailments, not just psoriasis. The major ailments for which saffron tea is considered beneficial include psoriasis, lacerations, eliminations, incoordination of assimilations and eliminations, toxemia, and ulcers.

From this list we can safely assume that saffron acts on the stomach and intestines and helps alleviate skin aliments caused by a malfunction in the alimentary canal.

Preparation of Saffron Tea (as my patients are directed):

In the evening or just before retiring—

Place a quarter teaspoon of saffron tea in a cup then pour boiling water over it. Allow to stand fifteen to thirty minutes. Strain, cool, and drink. This should be made fresh each time. This tea should be taken consistently, at least until all the lesions have healed.

Note that it is best taken at night, just before retiring. Some patients report that they enjoy having a few cups during the day as well. The most beneficial effects of the tea are that of flushing out the liver and kidneys, increasing perspiration, and promoting healing of the intestinal lesions. Saffron tea has also been called an intestinal antiseptic. It should be regarded as a valuable part of the therapeutic regimen. This tea is to be taken consistently until the skin is clear, and then periodically to keep the "passageways" cleansed for proper elimination.*

Saffron Water is a variant of Saffron Tea that can be helpful in severe cases of psoriasis. The idea is to have some saffron in all the drinking water. This would not be as concentrated as the tea, but its cleansing effect is without equal.

To one gallon of pure boiling water, add one teaspoon of American yellow saffron tea and allow the mixture to steep a few minutes. This will be just enough to give the water a yellowish tinge. When cool, strain the water and pour it into a glass or porcelain container(s) and place in a refrigerator. This is to be used as drinking water whenever desired. I recommend my patients drink at least four glasses a day. This may be considered part of the 6 to 8 glasses of drinking water suggested daily. In time, the cleansing effect of the saffron water will bring about beneficial results, provided the patient conforms to all other rules of the regimen.

---

*Readers who wish a more detailed account of the benefits of Saffron Tea are advised to purchase *An Edgar Cayce Health Anthology* which includes a comprehensive article, "The Healing Powers of Saffron Tea" by Robert O. Clapp and may be ordered from the A.R.E. Bookstore, Box 595, Virginia Beach, VA 23451.

There have been occasions when a patient developed the sensation in the bladder of a desire to urinate even when the bladder had recently been emptied. This can be attributed to the cleansing effect of the saffron tea. After a period of time, in flushing out the kidneys, it causes a constant flow of urine into the bladder to be voided. The patient begins urinating more often than he or she is used to, causing the inner lining of the bladder to wear down somewhat, especially in the area of the sphincter trigone at the bottom of the bladder. This in turn causes stimulation of the stretch fibers, giving the sensation that one has to urinate, but the patient finds it not necessary and wonders what may be happening. One patient was advised to have his kidneys X-rayed and his prostate checked, when all that proved necessary was to take him off the saffron tea for a couple of weeks. As a result, the condition cleared up promptly.

Saffron Vapor can be useful in dealing with psoriasis on the face. Although it appears less frequently on the face and hands, there are many cases in which psoriasis breaks out in these areas. This can cause considerable anxiety in the patient since, obviously, these areas are highly visible. Exposure of the head and hands to the rays of the sun undoubtedly helps keep these areas relatively clear of the lesions, but when this is not enough, some of my patients have succeeded in clearing facial psoriasis by steeping some saffron or camomile tea in a basin of hot water, then placing a towel over the head and leaning over the basin, allowing the steam to gently stimulate the skin. The procedure is similar to using Vicks VapoRub steam to break up a cold in the head.

Obviously, the flame under the pot should be extinguished because if the steam is too hot, the face can be scalded. The steam should be just warm and steady. One patient in particular had excellent results when, after the steam, she rubbed castor oil into the lesions, leaving it on overnight. As early as the next morning, after washing her face with cuticura soap, she saw a noticeable improvement.

The real clearing, however, still comes from the generalized internal cleansing of the body. This proved to be true in this case when the patient realized that the steam treatment was, at best, only temporary. She then drank a half gallon of saffron water over a period of a few hours. Urination was extremely frequent because of this measure, but *within one day* her face was practically one hundred percent clear! She attributes this remarkable result to the large quantity of saffron water she consumed. A general "flushing" of the liver and kidneys took place and helped drain the body of accumulated toxins. Today, her face is always as clear as she wants it to be.

Slippery Elm Bark Tea (ulmus fulva)

In his book *On Writing Well*, William Zinsser describes a particular display on view at the National Baseball Museum and Hall of Fame in Cooperstown, New York. It is a piece of slippery elm bark from Clear Lake, Wisconsin, birthplace of pitcher Burleigh Grimes. During the games, Grimes chewed this kind of bark "to increase saliva for throwing the spitball. When wet, the ball sailed to the plate in deceptive fashion".[1]

Now, unless you are a totally committed baseball buff, you would probably agree with Zinsser that "this would seem to be one of the least interesting facts available in America today." If, however, you are psoriatic, when you read the following account of another effective use of slippery elm bark the substance takes on a new significance.

Several years ago, the *A.R.E. News*, which is regularly sent to each member of the Association for Research and Enlightenment, published a report in its "Health and Beauty" column on the success of treatments for psoriasis based on Edgar Cayce's readings. The report noted that "some of the most heartwarming" stories of health regained through the readings were "those telling about the cure and control of psoriasis, often after many years of fruitless searching for a cure," and continued:

Mrs. B.C. of North Carolina writes that last summer after joining the A.R.E.:

"I obtained the Circulating File, Skin: Psoriasis. My fourteen-year old son had been afflicted with this ailment for six years and had fifty-cent-size patches on his scalp as well as elbows and stomach. From the psoriasis file I learned that this disease is caused mostly by the thinning of the walls of the intestinal tract, allowing toxins to leak into the circulatory system.

"Following suggestions from the readings, I put a pinch of ground elm bark into a glass of water and stirred it, letting the solution stand at least three minutes before drinking. I gave this to him once a day, and in ten days all traces of the psoriasis were gone and have not returned. To be on the safe side he continues to have his elm bark drink with his dinner each night."

Mrs. B.C.'s letter indicates that she allowed the slippery elm bark drink to stand for three minutes before serving it to her son. This agrees with Cayce's suggestion which states that slippery elm should be prepared about two to three minutes before it is drunk. It should not, however, be taken after it has stood for more than twenty or thirty minutes. We can safely assume therefore, that the drink should be taken anywhere from three to twenty minutes after preparation but under no circumstances should it be taken after standing for more than thirty minutes. Beyond that time it may become rancid.

Although Mrs. B.C. continued to give her son slippery elm with his dinner, best results are obtained by taking it first thing in the morning if possible one-half hour before breakfast. The saffron tea, on the other hand, is taken in the evening.

The next patient discussed in the A.R.E. News report, though requiring a fuller program of treatment, achieved the same amazing results in just as short a period of time. Mrs. M., the head of nursing in an Australian hospital, flew to the A.R.E. Clinic in Phoenix, Arizona with her husband after reading a book about Cayce. Having suffered with psoriasis for over fourteen years, Mrs. M. was overcome with joy at her almost completely clear skin after just two weeks of a Cayce-inspired course of treatment which included spinal adjustments, a special diet, and the herb drinks.

Having covered her blemished arms with long sleeves for all those years, Mrs. M. delightedly held out smooth, clear arms for our inspection.

"It's wonderful to be able to wear short-sleeved frocks again. And for the first time in four years," she added happily, "I'm wearing one pair of hose instead of two. Even going bare-legged!"

Stories such as these abound in the Virginia Beach library's circulating files. Mrs. B.C.'s story, the first case mentioned, held special interest for me in that apparently the only measure reportedly taken by her son was a pinch of ground elm bark in a glass of water once a day. Here at least is one case on record that proves the efficacy of slippery elm in the treatment of psoriasis, even when used alone.

The Chinese have long enjoyed the many benefits of slippery elm. They considered it one of nature's most excellent demulcents and nutritives, and employ it for its ability to absorb foul gases in the body, for its gentle, soothing action in cases of enteritis (inflammation of the intestinal tract) and colitis (inflammation of the large bowel) and because its soothing, mucilaginous nature makes bowel evacuation easier and more effective.[2]

From these accounts, as well as the Chinese influence, we can conclude that the slippery elm acts as a protective coating along the inner lining of the upper and lower intestinal tract. This can not only prevent seepage of toxins, but helps the healing process of the thin, porous intestinal walls as well as aid in evacuation.

Ileitis and Psoriasis: A Connecting Link?

It has been brought to my attention that several patients suffering from ileitis (inflammation of the intestines) have shown tendencies toward developing psoriasis. This is especially noted in cases where the ileitis is severe. Doctors connected with research in ileitis feel there is a link between the two diseases but cannot come up with an explanation. In the light of what has been presented thus far in this treatise, a possible cause seems to evolve. If the theory I have been working on is correct; namely, a "seepage" of toxins permeates the intestinal walls thereby invading the lymph and blood circulatory system, then anything that causes the intestinal walls to break down can in turn cause that same seepage to take place rendering the patient prone to septicemia or toxic build-up in the blood. Psoriasis, or other dermatologic problems would naturally follow as the body attempts to rid itself of accumulated poisons. Ileitis, especially if severe, most certainly compromises the intestinal walls, thus strengthening what I consider to be a reasonable explanation for connecting the two diseases. Perhaps it would be well for western researchers to consider using slippery elm in cases of ileitis. The Chinese have used it successfully for centuries.

Preparation of Slippery Elm drink (as my patients are directed):

Instructions for preparing slippery elm bark are quite specific and should be followed implicitly:

Place about a quarter teaspoon of slippery elm bark powder in a cup of *warm* water. Stir and let stand about fifteen minutes before drinking. Again, do not let it stand beyond thirty minutes as it may become rancid. This mixture is taken in the early morning, at least one half hour before breakfast if possible, for the first ten days of the regimen. It is then reduced to every other day, except in severe cases, until the skin condition clears.

Most people have no problem swallowing the slippery elm drink, but if it is difficult to get down, adding ice to the mixture is suggested.

Slippery Elm Bark is also available and may be chewed. For some people this is no problem, but most find it not only difficult to do but unsightly as well. A more palatable and convenient alternative is to obtain Thayer's Slippery Elm lozenges in a health food store or a well supplied drug store. Taking a few of these a day usually serves the same purpose.

The importance of taking saffron and slippery elm, especially in severe or stubborn cases, cannot be overemphasized. These herbal teas effect the gastric flow throughout the stomach and stimulate the walls of the intestinal tract to bring about healing of the distressed areas.

Our approach to alleviating psoriasis, remember, is primarily based on diet and healing the intestinal walls and insuring adequate evacuation. Slippery elm bark powder, in the form of teas or chewables, taken regularly, is a vital part of this healing process which I consider mandatory *with one important exception*:

IF A WOMAN WITH PSORIASIS IS PREGNANT, OR EXPECTS TO BE, SLIPPERY ELM IS *NOT* RECOMMENDED. IT HAS BEEN IMPLICATED IN CAUSING MISCARRIAGE. (Hochner, *Pregnancy & Childbirth* Avon Books).

NOTE: A patient may, if desired, reverse the order in which Saffron Tea and Slippery Elm is taken. In other words, the Saffron may be taken in the morning, while the Slippery Elm is taken at night; the object being that they are not taken too close to each other as this would nullify their effect.

Camomile Tea (anthemis nobilis):

Camomile tea is one of the oldest and best known home remedies which grows abundantly almost everywhere. Most health food stores are well supplied with this tea. Camomile tea may be used as an occasional alternate to Saffron because it is believed that the two herbs work similarly on the body.

Numerous benefits have been attributed to camomile, including the alleviation of kidney, bronchial, and bladder problems and even bruises and sprains when camomile and bittersweet, as an ointment, are combined (Kloss)[3]. The most widely recognized use of camomile by herbalists, however, is as a tonic for the body. It is also one of the most aromatic and pleasant-tasting teas available.

As mentioned earlier, some of my patients with psoriatic lesions on their faces were pleasantly surprised with good results when they steeped saffron and allowed the gentle fumes to rise up, engulfing the face. This procedure was also used with a measure of success by using camomile in the same fashion.

Although camomile tea was often recommended, saffron tea should be taken more frequently. Camomile tea should be prepared in the same way as saffron.

Mullein Tea (verbascoum thapsus):

Mullein is the fourth herb tea specifically suggested for psoriasis. Fresh leaves for the making of tea are preferred, if available; if not, dry leaves will suffice. Mullein tea should begin after slippery elm tea has been taken for about ten days.

Preparation for Mullein Tea:

Crumble or crush a *teaspoon* of mullein leaves and place in a cup. Pour a pint of *boiling* water over it and allow it to steep for thirty minutes. Strain, cool, and drink, not necessarily all at once, but over the course of three or four hours.

Note that in the case of mullein tea, a full teaspoon should be used and the brew should stand for thirty minutes before drinking. It should also be noted that mullein, and in fact *all* the herbs for making the teas discussed in this chapter, should always be stored in a refrigerator. If they aren't, they may become "buggy," especially in the summer, even if packaged properly.

Watermelon Seed Tea (citrullus vulgaris):

Last, but not least, Watermelon Seed Tea has been known for its effectiveness as a diuretic and has been credited for helping bladder infections for centuries. I suggest this tea to my patients as a substitute for Saffron as an aid in flushing out the urinary system.

Preparation for Watermelon Seed Tea:

Two tablespoons of the tea are boiled for five minutes in a pint of water. It is then covered and allowed to stand until cold before drinking. One cup, three or four times a day is suggested.

Watermelon Seed Tea is available commercially in the form of loose tea or in tea bags.

In conclusion, I advise my patients to persist in taking the herb teas as directed, and to have confidence that by doing so they will be taking a major step in the alleviation of psoriasis.

<u>NOTE</u>: The herb teas mentioned in this chapter are available at most well-supplied health food stores, or they may be ordered through the Cayce product suppliers listed in Appendix C.

REFERENCES

(Chapter 7—Herb Teas)

1. William Zinsser, *On Writing Well*, (New York, NY, pub. Harper & Row, copyright 1976), p. 55.
2. Richard Lucas, *Secrets of the Chinese Herbalists*, (West Nyack, NY, pub. Parker Publishing Co., Inc., copyright 1977), pp. 191-192.
3. Jethro Kloss, *Back to Eden*, (New York, NY, pub. Laurer Books, Inc., copyright 1971), pp. 212-213.

The Role of the Spine

The role the spine plays in the phenomenon of psoriasis is far more profound than ordinarily assumed. The following chapter, dealing with the spine and its neural connections, may seem a bit technical for the average reader. I hope, however, that it will help others, especially professionals, to understand why manual adjustments of the spine are an important part of the therapy suggested in the Edgar Cayce works.

It is my purpose to answer the questions of both lay and professional readers as simply, yet thoroughly, as possible. The following information, I trust, will encourage active use of spinal adjustments whenever possible by showing that the reasoning behind them is solidly founded on scientific facts.

Chapter 8

The Role of the Spine

If it is difficult for you to see the connection between the spinal column and skin diseases, you are not alone. For a long time I did not appreciate their interrelation myself, and neither did most of my chiropractic colleagues and medical friends. Our attitude was that we should leave the skin to the dermatologists, the bones to the orthopedists, and manipulations of the spine to the osteopaths or chiropractors. On the surface this concept looks reasonable and has been more or less the accepted way of healing in this age of specialization. However, it can be carried to unreasonable extremes, as the following story illustrates.

A well-established physician and a young medical student about to graduate were having a conversation regarding today's tendency to compartmentalize:

Student: "Doctor, I appreciate the time you are giving me before I enter practice."

Doctor: "You're welcome. Are you going to enter general practice?"

Student: "No, I decided to specialize."

Doctor: "Eye, Ear, Nose and Throat?"

Student: "Well, no, I decided to specialize in the nose only."

Doctor: "Oh, really? Ah—which nostril?"

A new consciousness that recognizes the oneness of all things is now emerging. This idea of "oneness," in itself, is really not new it has been discussed and respected since the days of Paracelsus, Hippocrates and Pythagoras but the concept is being rekindled in our present age and is often referred to as "holism." As mentioned earlier, when it is applied to health care, we speak of "holistic medicine." Granted, without a basic understanding of the body's mechanisms, it is next to impossible to appreciate the plausibility of the holistic view of health and disease. Pottenger's *Symptoms of Visceral Disease* states: "Diseases cannot be divided into those of this and that organ; for the human body is a unit. One part cannot be diseased without affecting other parts. No organ can be understood except in its relationship to other organs and to the body as a whole."[1] These principles are the foundation-stones of the holistic approach to healing.

It is readily understood, not only among physicians, but also by a large segment of the general public, that the nervous system controls the various functions of the body. Should the nervous system not function properly, the whole body or some part of it will feel the effects to a greater or lesser degree. This is basic physiology—an incontrovertible law.

Since our ultimate goal is to get to the root causes of the disease and our theory involves the integrity of the walls of the intestinal tract, it behooves us to at least investigate its neural connections, that is, where they originate and what may possibly happen if the normal nerve impulses are altered.

The upper intestinal tract is supplied by nerve impulses emanating from the mid-dorsal vertebrae (the area located between the shoulder blades). If these nerve roots are traumatized by say, direct injury, curvature of the spine or *subluxations* (misaligned vertebrae), the normal flow of nerve energy may be disturbed. In fact, one discourse by Cayce clearly states that even one subluxation can cause psoriasis by the effect an impinged nerve or nerves would have on the normal blood circulation to the walls of portions of the intestinal tract. Normal circulation would be impaired thus causing an impoverishment of these walls which leads to their eventual breakdown. This, in turn, will render them more permeable to toxic elements. The thinning of the intestinal walls is not only conceivable, but predictable. The intestinal walls can become so porous on a microscopic level, that "seepage" of toxic elements can readily find their way into the lymphatics and bloodstream by a process of osmosis. If this "poisoning" is not counteracted, the kidneys and liver the major filtering systems of the body become overtaxed and the body calls into play its next "backup" system, the skin, to eliminate the toxins—hence the outward manifestation of psoriasis.

The principle that abnormal digestive tract nerve impulses can cause disease apparently holds true not only for psoriasis and other skin problems, but for many of the degenerative ailments as well. For instance, in the discourses on multiple sclerosis, Cayce frequently referred to the cause as being the body's inability to *assimilate gold* into the system. Why would anyone be unable to assimilate gold? For one of two reasons: either not enough gold is supplied by the diet or, more plausibly, the body cannot absorb the gold even if it is adequately supplied. (Foods considered to have a high gold content are Salsify [Oyster Plant], Carrots, and Shellfish.) Assuming food intake is adequate, the next question is obvious. Why is a food absorbed or not absorbed? William A. McGarey, M.D., in an article based on the Cayce material, answers as follows:

> "The physiological progression of events, as seen in the readings, seems to be fairly consistent. There is either an "acid" condition developed within the body as a result of infection of a chronic nature (which has its terminal effect on the liver, pancreas and spleen) or an autonomic nervous system malfunction in the *mid-dorsal region from D4 to D9** which affects the functioning of the liver or directly upsets the normal activity in the stomach when digestion starts. Improper functioning of the liver, pancreas and spleen in turn creates `used, refused energies' in the circulatory system, and these in turn *suppress assimilation* of necessary food substances in the lacteal duct area of the small intestine."[2]

Altered nerve impulses from the spine to the digestive tract evidently can cause these effects in the same way that other abnormalities can result in the digestive tract from spinal misalignment and bring about a condition of psoriasis or other dermatological problems. Diseases may have different names and affect us in different ways without necessarily having different causes. The "autonomic nervous system malfunction"

---

*D4 to D9 refers to the section of the spine extending from the 4th Dorsal (or Thoracic) to the 9th Dorsal vertebrae.

Dr. McGarey speaks of may very well mean vertebrae out of their proper alignment, known professionally as subluxations.

Your Spine

To study the intricate workings of the spine is to delve into a marvel of living architecture and function. Each vertebra is positioned perfectly in relation to every other to provide both maximum strength and a flexibility that sometimes, as in the case of dancers, comes close to simulating the movements of a snake. This places the human spine in the category of a biological engineering miracle. Add to this the spine's primary function of protecting the "lifeline" of the body, the spinal cord, and you begin to see the capabilities of a human mechanism that scientists estimate took 100 million years to evolve.

Of the 206 bones in the adult skeleton, 33 comprise the backbone or spinal column. These 33 are known as the vertebrae. In comparison to other bones, the vertebrae are considered small, but their purpose is anything but small. These 33 separate and distinct, highly engineered bones are separated into five divisions. The smallest bones are the *cervical (neck) vertebrae* which allow their division a wider range of motion than the rest of the spine. The *dorsal (or thoracic) vertebrae* are 12 in number and make up the upper back; they begin at just below the 7th cervical vertebrae. Heavier than the cervical vertebrae, the dorsals also hold the ribs in place at junctions called *articular facets*, special disc-shaped indentations. The next five vertebrae are located in the lower back. Called the *lumbar vertebrae*—they bear most of the body's weight.

The position of each facet on each vertebra, relative to the next, plays a major role in what is termed a *vertebral subluxation* or *vertebral lesion* (mentioned earlier).

There are four distinct curves in the adult spine. At birth, however, there is only one continuous curve, a generalized convex or *kyphotic* curve. After birth, as the child begins to develop and bend his or her neck, the cervical curve, concave or *lordotic* begins to appear. A similar process occurs in the lower back, forming the concave curve of the lumbar spine. The four distinct spinal curves are featured in the following illustration. Note that I have specifically pointed out the 6th and 7th dorsal (thoracic), 3rd cervical, 9th dorsal and 4th lumbar vertebrae. These are the vertebral segments that are directly involved in combating psoriasis due to their neural connections.

THE SPINE:

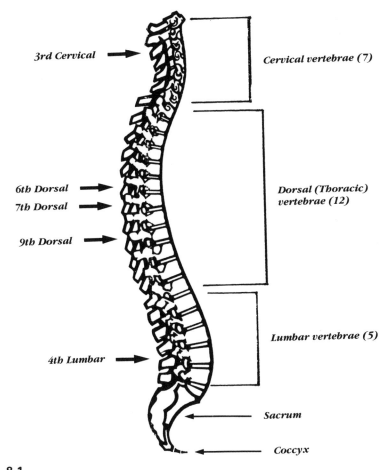

Fig. 8-1

Reprinted by permission: Chiropractic Public Relations (CPR), 141 Blauvelt Street, Teaneck, NJ 07666.

Beneath the lumbar vertebrae is the *sacrum,* which at birth is really five separate smaller vertebrae that finally fuse at about age twenty-five to form a wedgeshaped bone which fits between the two hip bones. Beneath the sacrum, at the very end of the spine, is the *coccyx,* known as the tail bone. This, too, begins as separate small bones (four in number) which fuse into one in the adult.

Between each of the cervical, thoracic and lumbar vertebrae and between the fifth lumbar and the sacrum are specialized cushions, *the intervertebral discs*. These discs, which make up about 25 percent of the adult's spine length, are designed to absorb shock and keep the bones from grinding against each other. They also permit greater flexibility between the vertebrae and allow for changes in body balance. Being relatively soft and flexible, they easily adapt to changes in posture. By separating one vertebra from another, the discs also provide openings which allow the nerves that emerge from the spinal cord to pass, unobstructed, between the vertebrae. The openings, *the intervertebral foramina*, can be altered in size and shape to an abnormal degree by injury, poor posture, spinal defects, or idiopathic (unknown) causes. Such changes in one of the openings can cause a pressure point and/or an inflammation of nerve roots located at that opening. The chiropractic theory of health and disease holds that this condition, referred to as a subluxation, is a major cause of abnormal states in the body that can result in a wide range of symptoms, from pain to abnormal physiological function. Osteopaths use the term *spinal lesion* to describe essentially the same thing. The treatment in both professions is also basically the same—spinal adjustment or manipulation, an ancient art, to relieve the pressure point.

SPINAL SUBLUXATION:

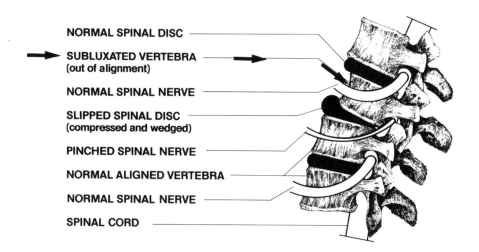

NORMAL SPINAL DISC

SUBLUXATED VERTEBRA
(out of alignment)

NORMAL SPINAL NERVE

SLIPPED SPINAL DISC
(compressed and wedged)

PINCHED SPINAL NERVE

NORMAL ALIGNED VERTEBRA

NORMAL SPINAL NERVE

SPINAL CORD

Fig. 8-2

Reprinted by permission: Chiropractic Public Relations (CPR), 141 Blauvelt Street, Teaneck, NJ 07666

At this point, to go into specific anatomical, neural connections between the spinal cord and the intestinal tract would serve no useful purpose in this edition. Such concise, detailed information is being considered for a professional volume in the future. Suffice it here to simply state that the nerve supply to the upper intestinal tract, in particular the areas of the duodenal-jejunal junction (flexure), originate in the mid-dorsal area of the spine; the sixth and seventh dorsals being the principal vertebrae involved.

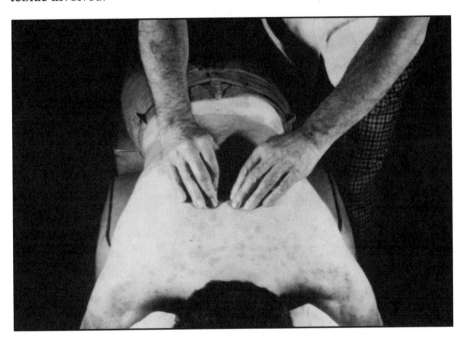

Fig. 8-3
Palpation of the 6th and 7th Dorsal Vertebrae

Further confirmation of the neural connections between the spinal cord and the digestive and emunctory organs may be found in *Pathogenesis of Visceral Disease Following Vertebral Lesions*, a study published by the American Osteopathic Association after extensive research. One chapter, "Gastrointestinal Changes Following Lesions," concludes in part (from experiments on animals) that lesions of the "seventh and eighth, probably also the sixth, ninth and tenth" thoracic vertebrae were "followed by lowered strength, diminished elasticity and increased extensibility of the muscular walls of the stomach and intestines".[3] In simpler terms, the researchers found that such lesions or subluxations apparently compromised the intestinal walls that, in theory at least, play a major role in the cause of psoriasis, thus strengthening the Cayce concept.

The reason for also concentrating on the 3rd Cervical, 9th Dorsal and 4th Lumbar is because these are the areas of the spine where lymph centers and their neural and circulatory connections are disturbed.

Innervation of the Skin

Can spinal adjustments conceivably aid the skin *directly* as well as revitalizing the internal organs that eliminate waste and neutralize toxins? I contend that they can and do, particularly general, full-spine adjustments.

The skin is actually an organ, in fact, the largest organ of the body. Every cell in every organ of the human body must receive electrical (nerve) energy to remain in a state of health, and this organ is no exception. There is indeed a nerve supply to the skin itself, and as Pottenger states, "The structures of the skin, as far as physiologists have been able to determine, possess only sympathetic nerves receiving innervation from the thoracic (dorsal) and upper three lumbar segments".[4]

Therefore, from the first dorsal down to the third lumbar, a total of 15 vertebral segments, there is a relationship between the spine and the structures of the skin by way of the nerves that emanate from between these vertebrae. Owing to this anatomical/physiological fact, spinal adjustments can indeed benefit dermal structures, whether or not a skin disease is actually present.

Contradictions?

Several questions will probably occur to you regarding apparent contradictions in what I have said so far: First, that psoriasis is caused by a thinning of the upper intestinal walls; second, that it is due to chronic constipation; third, that poor diet is to blame; and now, that something is out of alignment in the spine. Can all these statements be equally valid? Is there any one cause that is common to all cases?

It should be understood that these different causes of psoriasis can work in conjunction with one another. the *only* apparent common denominator among psoriatics is that, for one reason or another, *the patient cannot handle the toxic buildup produced in his or her body*. The organs that normally eliminate toxins fail to do the job effectively and thus the skin, the body's final line of defense, is pressed into service.

If we look upon psoriasis as a *condition* rather than a specific disease, we will stop looking for *the* cause and seriously examine the *causes*. It is up to the treating physician to determine why the patient builds up toxins. When he solves that riddle, he can proceed intelligently in recommending therapy. More often than not, good results will follow given adequate time.

The Spinal Adjustment: Rationale and Technique

When people think of having a spinal adjustment administered by a competent chiropractor or osteopath, it is usually because pain is present in some area of the spine. This is well and good because, in the vast majority of such cases, an adjustment is just what is needed and, most likely, will clear up the problem if misaligned vertebrae are the basic cause.

Rarely, however, do people realize that a spinal adjustment may be needed in connection with the actual *function* of specific organs particularly those of the abdominal viscera, because there is often no telltale sign of pain when one or more of these organs is not functioning properly. There may be other signs, to be sure, such as jaundice, malaise, or headache, but people do not readily connect these symptoms with the spine. This, I believe, is one reason why some patients cannot appreciate the benefits of spinal adjustments in relation to psoriasis. They are more versed in being treated for pain by a chiropractor or osteopath than in having these practitioners make spinal adjustments to release nerve energy needed for proper functioning of the abdominal organs. A quick reference to accepted textbooks on anatomy and physiology will confirm the wisdom that spinal adjustments can play a *major* role in psoriasis therapy. The beneficial effect they may have on the digestive tract, the alimentary canal, the glandular centers, and the skin itself warrants serious consideration.

As the techniques of spinal adjustment have evolved over the years, new and innovative methods have appeared in both the osteopathic and chiropractic fields. My own profession, chiropractic, has introduced an array of reflex techniques, newly designed manipulative tables, traction devices, and instruments, all developed to help maintain or restore the integrity of the spine. However, in my opinion, the preferred methods of spinal manipulation are the traditional, time-honored, proved techniques first promulgated by D.D. Palmer in chiropractic and A.J. Still in osteopathy. Contact and angle of thrust are made directly on the spine, with particular attention to the 6th and 7th dorsal vertebrae and the 3rd cervical, 9th dorsal and 4th lumbar. The manipulator (chiropractor or osteopath) who does not effectively adjust these areas is falling short of the mark and is of no service to the patient.

Trying to prove that a subluxation existed often ends in frustration, for in many cases, it cannot be demonstrated clinically. It can, however, be assumed. Whether a patient responds favorably or not is all that really matters and, quite frankly, all the patient cares about. J.F. Bourdillon, past president of the North American Academy of Manipulative Medicine and former consultant orthopedic surgeon to the Gloucestershire Royal Hospital in England, effectively reminds us in his book *Spinal Manipulation* that practical results, rather than scientific analysis, have always been the main aim of physicians. Our modern preoccupation with science makes us too easily forget that "only a few generations ago medicine was an art, and the large majority of medical and surgical treatment was based on the results of practical experience rather than on firm scientific foundation".[5]

How Effective are Adjustments?

Why is the spinal adjustment so vital to the psoriatic? Because it can not only help restore the normal integrity of the intestinal wall that is essential to an alleviation of the condition, but it can also make possible the one thing a psoriatic is most interested in—*a permanent cure*. If the entire psoriatic syndrome has its *origin* in spinal subluxations, correcting these subluxations should be the first line of attack against the disease. It is my conclusion therefore, according to logic and theory, that if one has the required adjustments of the spine and follows through with all the other measures called for in the regimen, a permanent cure is possible.

Only time and further research can provide the final answer regarding permanence of the cure. One thing, however, is certain in following this alternative approach—if successful, the patient knows that he or she is then permanently in control of the condition.

We can more easily appreciate the role spinal adjustments have in the treatment of psoriasis when we read Pottenger's explanation of the significance of the nervous system in maintaining the harmonious, integrated functioning of every cell and organ of the body:

"Each body cell has its own action and each organ its own function. If each cell or organ should function without regard to other cells or organs, it would be equivalent to all citizens of a state living and acting without regard for others. A state of anarchy would result. Harmonious activity can come only through correlation of action. In the animal organism this correlation is brought about partly through chemical substances but mainly through the nervous system, as previously mentioned. Through it the action of every cell is subordinated to the good of the whole".[6]

Such considerations, I believe, lead to only one conclusion—*manipulation of the spine helps maintain the all-important coordinating function of the nervous system.* It is, therefore, conceivable that a person suffering from psoriasis can benefit from spinal manipulations by virtue of the fact that the intestinal tract, as well as the structure of the skin itself, is supplied by nerve impulses emanating from the dorsal spine.

"Look well to the spine for the cause of disease"—Hippocrates.

In summary, then, the primary areas of the spine to be adjusted are illustrated below.

ADJUSTMENTS OF THE SPINE:

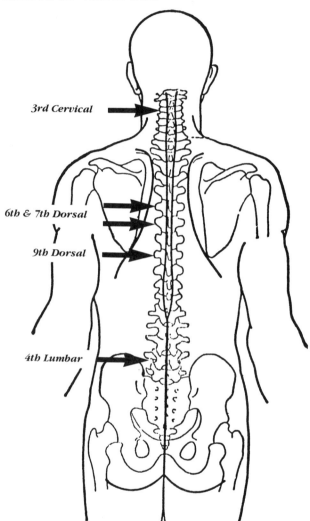

Fig. 8-4

Basic illustration from Gray's Anatomy, 26th ed. (Philadelphia, Lea & Febiger, 1954). Reprinted by permission. (30th Edition, Pub. in 1985, Edited by Carmine D. Clemente.) Labeled by the author.

REFERENCES

(Chapter 8—The Role of the Spine)

1. Francis Marion Pottenger, *Symptoms of Visceral Disease*, ed. 7, (St. Louis, 1953, The C.V. Mosby Co.) p. 9.
2. William A. McGarey, M.D., Article "Indigestion," *Health Care Report* Vol. 1 No. 4, pub. The Edgar Cayce Foundation, Virginia Beach, VA.
3. *Pathogenesis of Visceral Disease Following Vertebral Lesions* (Chicago, IL, pub. by the American Osteopathic Association, 1948) p. 232.
4. Pottenger, p. 410.
5. J.F. Bourdillon, *Spinal Manipulation* (London, William Heinemann Medical Books Ltd. and Appleton-Century-Crofts, New York, ed. 3, 1982) p. 2.
6. Pottenger, p. 42.

Chapter 9

External Applications

The most important thing to grasp about external (topical) applications is that *all* of them are but palliative. As effective as some of them are in soothing the inflamed skin of psoriasis, they do not get to the root cause of the disease. The oils and ointments make the skin more pliable, rendering it less prone to splitting and cracking, which is a major problem for many psoriasis sufferers. Removal of scales and less new scaling seems to be a fringe benefit when using these creams and oils. Personally, I believe they aid in healing the surface cells by acting therapeutically on the lesions as if they were wounds.

No one can deny that both the sun and ultraviolet light treatments have often helped alleviate surface lesions and kept some patients clear for several months. An equal number, however, have experienced the pain and discouragement of their lesions returning, often worse than before. The obvious reason for their return is that the root cause of the disease is not affected by surface applications. Nevertheless, the following measures suggested for the purpose of soothing the surface areas can alleviate at least some of the distressing symptoms, particularly itching. They can allay the condition while the basic internal cause is being corrected. My patients choose those that work best for them by simple trial and error. I have mentioned only those that are practical in application as well as readily available.

1. Olive Oil/Peanut Oil Mixture

2. Castor Oil

3. Cuticura soap, Ointment, and Shampoo

4. Resinol

5. Carbolated Vaseline and Baker's P&S Liquid

6. Epsom Salts Baths

7. Fume and/or Steam Baths

8. Sunlight and Ultraviolet Light

9. Sodium Bicarbonate (Baking Soda) and Aveeno Baths

10. Witch Hazel—Listerine—Glyco-Thymoline

11. Electrical Stimulation and Ultrasound

12. Camphorated Oil

13. Olive Oil/Tincture of Myrrh Mixture

14. Hydrophilic Ointment

15. Physiotherapy Units for home use

Olive Oil/Peanut Oil Mixture

A mixture of equal parts olive oil and peanut oil is one of the most soothing applications when massaged into individual lesions or over the entire body. It also helps prevent the cracking of dried lesions. This mixture is most useful in the winter when the humidity in a home or apartment is low due to artificial heat. It is also the best application for the scalp when a vise-like feeling grips the patient's head and lesions characterized by a white, snow-capped appearance, as well as "lumps" are seen or felt all over the scalp.

I suggest the use of the olive oil/peanut oil mixture more than any other external oil application at home because, as mentioned, it helps heal the surface cells, enhances the skin's pliability, and is relatively easy to clean when applied to the scalp. This is detailed in my chapter, "The Crowning Glory."

If the lesions are thick and disfiguring throughout the torso, I advise my patients to massage the mixture well into the lesions and then place a plastic bag, such as those used for dry-cleaning purposes, over the torso. An opening is cut for the head and two for the arms, then cut to waist length and worn underneath pajamas. In the morning, the plastic bag is removed and discarded. Plastic bags can be used on the thighs or legs as well, but not at the same time as the torso. There must be enough body surface exposed to the air for the skin to "breathe" efficiently. I emphasize extreme caution when and if this method is used on children, since plastic bags may accidentally cause strangulation or suffocation.

Two or three bag treatments a week are usually sufficient even in the most severe cases. Naturally, as the condition improves, this type of application can be cut down until it is no longer necessary.

A similar application may be used for the arms, particularly the elbows, the only difference being that plastic wrap is used instead of the bags to seal off the skin.

I have found this method to be a good substitute for the more elaborate occlusion suits used by some psoriatics. The plastic bags are simply discarded after use and cost practically nothing.

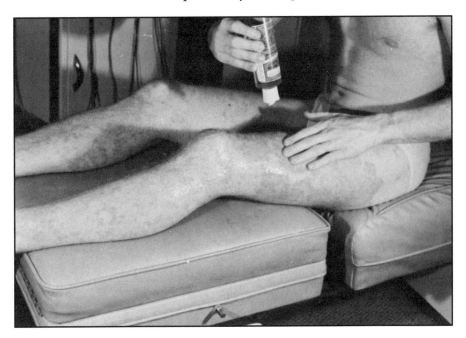

Fig. 9-1
Massaging an Olive Oil/Peanut Oil Mixture into the lesions

145

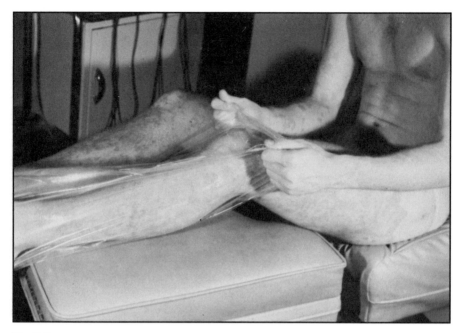

Fig. 9-2
Placing plastic wrap over the lesions after they were deeply massaged with the oils

Some patients have problems using plastic wrap or baggies directly over the skin. They find it to be too hot, sweaty and generally uncomfortable. Much more to their satisfaction is to simply eliminate the plastic or rubber wrappings and use only the cotton gloves, or socks directly over the hands or feet after they have been massaged with the castor oil or olive oil/peanut oil mixture. For large areas such as the back, chest or abdomen, they rub the oils in deeply, allow the oils to absorb for a few minutes, then put on a white cotton overshirt or sweat-shirt and retire for the night. Frankly, I prefer this to the age old method of using plastic or rubber wrapping directly over the oil. For one thing, it is much more comfortable. Add to that the fact that it allows the skin to breathe and is less restrictive. The difference, however, is obvious; it is not disposable. Laundering the garments after use would have to be made part of the routine. Patients have found, however, that the advantages of using white cotton-like garments, without the plastic wraps far outweigh the inconvenience of laundering.

A good washing tip to keep in mind when washing the oil stained clothing is to add a small box of Sodium Bicarbonate (Baking Soda) to the water during the wash cycle. It will help remove the oil from the garments. It goes without saying that the wash should contain only the clothes used for this purpose, even if it means accumulating them in their own hamper for a few days before washing. Realize that there will always be a certain amount of staining of the clothing or linens no matter how carefully they are washed, so obviously, patients should not use their best linens for this purpose.

The only drawback in applying the olive oil/peanut oil mixture is that the patient smells like a salad! However, presently on the market is an olive oil/peanut oil mixture with an almond scent that makes all the difference. It is available through Home Health Products and The Heritage Store, both located in Virginia Beach. (See Appendix C.)

Castor Oil

Castor oil has more benefits attributed to it than most people realize. Far from regarding it as only a natural cathartic when taken internally, castor oil is a most effective topical application for several conditions not normally associated with its use. I have successfully used it on warts, sprains, and strains in athletic injuries and even on myself when I had a kidney stone attack.

In psoriasis cases, castor oil should be viewed as a topical application to be used particularly on heavy, circumscribed lesions. (See case of J.R., Color Photo Section). The castor oil should be "Cold-Pressed, AA-USP" which is available through the Home Health Products and the Heritage Store. The best use of the oil is to gently rub it into the lesions, rather liberally, and to leave it on overnight or at least for several hours. Because of its viscosity (thickness) it is not used as a scalp treatment or for massaging the body in general as it would be rather difficult to remove. On smaller, circumscribed areas, however, it can be most effective.

There are certain combinations that increase the usefulness of the oil. Castor oil rubbed into a lesion, followed immediately by *Resinol,* applied right over the oil, helps relieve itching of the lesion. In the case of thickened heels and bottoms of the feet, castor oil combined with sodium bicarbonate (baking soda) and made into a paste and rubbed into thick, scaly heels or other heavily encrusted lesions, has shown remarkable results in most patients. If the skin is cracked, however, this combination may prove to be rather caustic and should not be used until the skin has

147

healed over. In such cases, the olive oil/peanut oil mixture or plain castor oil, without the baking soda, is used instead.

Cuticura Soap, Ointment, and Shampoo

Cuticura soap, ointment, and shampoo are among the oldest bath products available. This soap is widely used in cases of psoriasis when following my regimen. As mentioned earlier, the only time it is not used is if the patient has an allergic reaction because of some ingredient contained in its makeup which is rarely the case. Cuticura ointment has been very effective on large patches of psoriasis, particularly common vulgaris, which are well circumscribed and raised above the surface of the skin (acanthosis). It can be used alone or in combination with castor oil. A plastic wrapping over the lesion is needed to prevent soiling of clothing or linens as this compound is capable of heavy staining and discoloration. Mr. William Culmone, my first case described in Chapter 2, used cuticura ointment combined with castor oil extensively with excellent results. Cuticura shampoo is often effective on the scalp but may have to be ordered from a local druggist.

Resinol

Resinol is suggested to prevent itching. I have also found it quite helpful in combination with castor oil in the event Cuticura ointment is unavailable. Many new products to prevent itching are on the market these days, and I advise any patients to use whatever seems to help.

Carbolated Vaseline and Baker's P&S Liquid

These two products are used primarily along the hairline, on small circumscribed lesions of the scalp, and behind the ears. Although quite different in their makeup, they both have repeatedly proved to be helpful when used in these areas.

Carbolated vaseline is distinguished from the pure petroleum jelly by its brown appearance. Although it is used essentially along the hairline, it is not used extensively on the scalp in large areas because of the difficulty of washing it out. The hairline and the areas behind the ears where lesions often form usually respond well to this application. The substance should be applied preferably in the evening when gauze may be put over it to prevent soiling of linens. This same procedure applies to the Baker's P&S Liquid.

Epsom Salts Baths

An Epsom salts bath is one of the most beneficial, cleansing procedures readily available to most patients. The water should be comfortably hot and the tub filled enough so the patient's entire body, up to the neck, can be immersed. The water should contain about four pounds of Epsom salts. To use only a cup or two would not be very effective in most cases of psoriasis. I advise that the patient remain in the tub about twenty or thirty minutes, heating the water periodically as it cools. The water temperature is best kept at 106 degrees or 108 degrees Fahrenheit. If possible, these baths should be taken at least twice a week and followed with a good olive oil/ peanut oil massage before retiring for the night.

There are precautions, however, that must be observed. Epsom salts baths *should not* be taken if:

a. The patient has a heart or blood pressure problem;

b. The skin is cracked or is so sensitive that the salts cause a burning, painful sensation;

c. The patient is alone (in case of dizziness or faintness);

d. There is no one available to help the patient in or out of the tub should he or she be geriatric or severely arthritic.

The key word is CAUTION. Be sensible, don't be in a hurry. An Epsom salt bath should be one of the most soothing, gentle, cleansing procedures experienced by the psoriatic. My patients make it so when I insist they take the necessary precautions.

Fume or Steam Baths

This subject has already been adequately covered in my chapter on Internal Cleansing. It is merely listed here in that it may also be classified as an external application. In essence then, fume or steam baths may be thought of as an external application but one that aids internal cleansing. Therefore, I feel it is fitting to mention this procedure in both chapters.

Natural Sunlight

Natural sunlight is the best form of ultraviolet light for the psoriatic, but with two stipulations: never be exposed to the point of being sunburned, and never sunbathe between the hours of 11:00 A.M. and 3:00 P.M.

These precautions apply to *all* people, whether psoriatic or not, when one takes into account the warnings astronomers have issued in recent years about increased sunspot activity and the alarming destruction of our earth's protective ozone layer. More sunspot activity means more radioactive light coming into our atmosphere, leading to a higher incidence of skin cancer. So don't attempt to soak up too many "rays" in one sitting, even outside the midday hours.

Since some people are more sensitive to the sun's rays than others, we cannot say exactly how much is too much. Ten minutes could have little effect on one person and scald another. If a sunscreen is used in a lotion, it should be at least "15". There is also a decided difference between ten minutes on northern beaches, such as the North Atlantic Seaboard, and ten minutes in the tropical sun, such as the Caribbean. Gradual exposure is the safest way to go. Only time and experience can tell *you* what is right for you, but if it is a question of coming out of the sun sooner or later, make it sooner.

If areas of the skin do become burned I advise the application of Glyco-Thymoline, Apple cider vinegar diluted in water, or any of the known sunburn lotions that have proven to be helpful. Although apple cider vinegar diluted in water has been used successfully, I would not use it on open lesions. On areas where there are no lesions it may prove to be a godsend. It is best to try it on small areas first and observe the reaction. As always, caution is advised, as some individuals may react unfavorably.

It all boils down to exercising common sense. Patients particularly sensitive to the sun should avoid exposing their skin to it. However, ultraviolet light from the sun can still benefit psoriatics if they wear lightweight clothing. Even if not especially sensitive to the sun, patients should be careful not to overexpose themselves and, as mentioned, carefully choose the hours of the day to sunbathe. As a general rule: swimming in *clean* salt water, followed by *moderate* exposure to the sun is, in my opinion, the most beneficial external treatment available to the psoriatic.

Ultraviolet Light (Artificial)

Surprisingly, the external application of ultraviolet light has played a relatively minor role in the clearing of my patients' psoriasis. When they had an ultraviolet light home unit, I have not discouraged its use as long as it was prescribed by a dermatologist who gave proper instructions. Even under these conditions there can be dangers. On several occasions, the overuse of a patient's home unit caused a most severe reaction, marked by swollen eyelids, hypersensitive skin, and swollen lips which took several days to overcome.

Tanning parlors continue to gain in popularity throughout the United States, but again, the dangers involved should be clearly recognized. I do not encourage their continued use, if they must be used at all. I would like to call your attention to a June 17, 1985 Associated Press article entitled "AMA Cautions Against Tanning." This article clearly states, then as it does now, the latest medical view on the subject. Psoriatics and anyone else influenced by the public craze for tanning should take heed of its warnings:

"CHICAGO—The nation's largest organization of doctors is joining a growing chorus of medical voices condemning the pursuit of the perfect suntan.

There is no known medical benefit from cosmetic tanning, said a new report prepared for the American Medical Association's annual meeting, which began yesterday.

Although tanning lamps are advertised and sold as safer than earlier types, promising to provide tan without burning, sometimes even without protective goggles, is simply not true. Tanning in natural sunlight is also potentially dangerous, said the report, prepared by the AMA's Council on Scientific Affairs...The AMA's science council cited a recent study concluding that high-intensity, ultraviolet radiation emitted by even the newest and safest devices has no known beneficial effects to human health and is potentially dangerous. It said short-term and long-term exposure can cause changes in the skin, compromising its ability to ward off disease, causing it to degenerate and making it more likely to produce tumors. Exposure can also harm the eyes, damaging the retina and cause cataracts.

The American Cancer Society estimated last month that of the three main types of skin cancer, the deadly form, called malignant melanoma, is expected to develop in 22,000 Americans and kill 5,000 people this year—double the rate of ten years ago—mainly because of increased exposure to the sun."

For those who wish a more detailed discussion of ultraviolet light for home use, the National Psoriasis Foundation's 1981 Annual Report contains a full discussion of the subject in the chapter entitled "The ABC's of Ultra-Violet Light."*

Sodium Bicarbonate (Baking Soda) & Aveeno Baths

General itching, or pruritus, is one of the most irritating problems the psoriatic has to face, especially during the early stages of therapy. In many cases, about one pound of baking soda in a tub of comfortably hot water is very effective in relieving the itch. At times, I recommend two pounds in a tub of water. It may not work in every case, but it is inexpensive and certainly worth a try. A relatively new product on the market is Aveeno, which has an oatmeal base and is added to the tub of water. Results have been generally encouraging. This product is available in any drugstore. The idea is to find what works best for each patient and use it. A paste of sodium bicarbonate and apple cider vinegar often relieves the itch in circumscribed areas. The one thing a patient must *never* do is scratch it! The end result will only be increased irritation, bleeding, possible infection, and the formation of new psoriatic lesions.

[NOTE: I found it most interesting when at least one patient called to inform me of his almost immediate relief of generalized itching when he put *one* teaspoon of Sodium Bicarbonate in a glass of water and drank it. Within a few minutes after drinking it, the itch that was torturing him subsided. Undoubtedly, a shift in the chemistry of his body took place, rendering it more alkaline or at least neutralized the acidity throughout his system. Whatever the reason, the procedure was harmless but highly effective and may be helpful in some patients when generalized itching occurs.]

---

*National Psoriasis Foundation, 6415 S.W. Canyon Ct., Suite 200, Portland, Oregon 97221.

Witch Hazel—Listerine—Glyco-Thymoline

As an addition to the fume bath for psoriatics, *Witch Hazel,* as mentioned earlier, is used in this kind of hydrotherapy: A tablespoon of witch hazel is placed in half a pint of water that is used in the steam cabinet. In addition to helping to remove toxins, witch hazel placed in the waters of a fume bath provides another benefit—relief from itching. Sometimes, when all else fails, applying it directly to the irritated area proves helpful. It is applied with a cotton ball, or if there are no open cracks in the skin, the witch hazel can be applied directly with the fingers or palm of the hand.

Listerine, the popular throat antiseptic, is used primarily on areas on the scalp when itching is a problem. It is used by simply dabbing it on small lesions or diluted in warm water (about 20% Listerine to 80% water making one quart) and used as a general rinse following a shampoo.

Glyco-Thymoline is a red, alkaline mouth wash that has been on the market for many years. It may be ordered from a local druggist or from the suppliers listed in Appendix C. It too is applied directly to the skin to relieve itching or sunburn, as well as made into a diluted solution and used as a final rinse after a shampoo.

[NOTE: Glyco-Thymoline is one of those substances that has also been suggested as an alkalizer and intestinal antiseptic when taken internally. Most patients take just 4 or 5 drops in a glass of water before bedtime. It has been described in the Cayce material as an alimentary canal purifier, most desirable to the psoriatic and especially for those suffering from psoriatic arthritis. Patients usually take it five nights out of the week.]

Electrical Stimulation and Ultrasound

The *Electrical Stimulation* I speak of here refers to a physiotherapy unit, a muscle stimulator, applied only by a physician, to the primary areas of the spine directly involved in psoriasis; namely, the 3rd Cervical, 6th and 7th Dorsal, 9th Dorsal, and 4th Lumbar. (See Chapter "The Role of the Spine")

By applying small electrical pads to these specific areas, impulses may stimulate the nerve roots emanating from between these vertebrae helping to insure nerve flow to the glandular and internal organs that are involved. It is gentle in application, relaxing and, in general, may help the overall picture. This therapy, along with spinal adjustments and deep massage along the spine are the best natural methods I know of that can help insure normal nerve flow to the internal organs as well as the skin itself.

Ultrasound Heating (Controlled Hyperthermia): Studies conducted at Stamford University show that using ultrasound to heat the body helps clear the skin of psoriasis. This form of treatment is based simply on the fact that heat appears to benefit the psoriasis sufferers as is evident in the fact that psoriasis generally improves in the summer and gets worse in the winter. This therapy seems to work best on small, confined lesions.

I use it primarily in cases involving psoriasis of the palms of the hands. At times, the skin of the palms can become so thick with scales, stiffness, and cracking that it resembles elephant skin. The ultrasound, used with the patient's hands submerged in a basin of warm water, helps soften the heavily calloused palms which in turn allows an Oil/Electric Mitt home treatment to be more effective. (See Chapter, "Psoriasis on Hands and Feet"). This type of therapy should also be administered only by a physician or a trained staff member. It is mentioned here only for the benefit of those doctors who have access to an ultrasound unit but may not be aware of its effectiveness in such cases.

Camphorated Oil (Scar-Massage Formula)

Camphorated oil is a substance that has been on the medicinal market for many years. It has helped cure a multitude of ailments from chapped lips to laryngitis (it relieves the latter when applied as a hot pack over the throat). It has long served man well, that is, until recently. The Food and Drug Administration (FDA) banned the sale of camphorated oil because, as I understand it, too many people did not read instructions and took it internally. At the time of this writing it is unavailable in its pure form, but it is believed that it will probably come back under a new name.

Camphorated oil is suggested for removing some of the scars that may form as old psoriasis lesions heal. It is used for other types of scars as well, and is a major ingredient of the Cayce scar formula which is as follows:

Camphorated oil ....2 ounces
Lanolin (dissolved)...........................1/2 teaspoon
Peanut Oil (cold-pressed)..................1 ounce

This scar massage formula may be made up by the individual if and when camphorated oil is again available, or it may be purchased through the product suppliers listed in Appendix C. This combination can be effective in quickly halting the tendency to form a scar or scar tissue. I recommend rubbing this compound on scar-forming areas once a day, in amounts the skin will absorb. The eyes and mucous membranes are to be avoided. I do not hesitate to mention, however, that scars pose no apparent problem in many cases after healing is complete. For many patients, using the olive oil/peanut oil mixture was sufficient to cause the whitish scar areas to eventually disappear.

Olive Oil/Tincture of Myrrh Massage of the Abdomen

A thorough massage of the abdomen using a mixture of Olive Oil (heated) with an equal portion of Tincture of Myrrh can be one of the most beneficial measures a psoriatic patient can take. Concentrated kneading should take place, particularly along the right side of the abdomen. This is the area where congestion of fecal matter is most likely to occur. The action should be directed from below, upward along the right side to the lower right border of the rib cage—then left (slowly) across the stomach area to the left border of the abdomen—then down (slowly) along the left side to the pubic area. This action follows the normal path of the colon and will help move toxic accumulations (feces) out of the alimentary canal. If thorough enough, a massage once a week may be all that is necessary. Massaging slowly from right to left in a circular motion not only encourages peristaltic action of the colon but also helps stimulate circulation to the upper intestinal tract, the site of the thinning walls.

When my patients have no one available to give them the massage, I show them how to do it themselves. Lying on their back, knees up (to relax the abdomen), they follow the pattern just described. If a "sluggish" bowel is part of the problem, this type of massage will undoubtedly benefit the patient by enhancing his or her own eliminations.

Hydrophilic Ointment

In addition to the topical applications I already mentioned, Hydrophilic Ointment must be included in the list of creams that I have found to be quite consistent in soothing circumscribed lesions. It is simply rubbed into the lesion as is the cuticura ointment. However, there is no problem of staining. It must not be used near the eyes and, of course, should only be applied externally. It is a nonprescription item and may be obtained or ordered in any drugstore. I recommend my patients use the non-USP type which is soft and creamy (labeled "Differs from U.S.P."). I found this ointment to be quite effective on open lesions, but not on the "flexural" type of psoriasis where skin surfaces meet, such as underarms, breast folds, and gluteal crease. The ointment seems to irritate these areas since there is no air space.

The hydrophilic ointment, if hardened, can be made more "spreadable" and last longer by putting a full jar of it with half a jar of water in a mixing bowl. It is then whipped up with an electric mixer, using high speed, until the mixture has a consistency of shaving cream. It is then stored in a container large enough to hold the entire amount, or it is divided into smaller jars. In this form, the ointment can be used especially on large massive areas of the body and will more easily hold moisture. If the soft, creamy type is purchased, mixing is not necessary.

At first glance, all these applications and procedures may seem to be a lot of bother and difficult to remember. Actually, they are not. Once the ingredients are at my patient's fingertips and the measures are understood, the applications are quite simple to perform—with one additional benefit: the patient can do them at home at his own pace. It beats traveling to a psoriatic center, perhaps three or four times a week and probably some distance from home. The cost of these items is minimal and the possible side effects practically nonexistent. After a while, most patients find they do not need all these measures and can select the ones that best suit their particular condition and circumstances.

A Personal Observation

It is my contention that external applications help rid the body of lesions because the emulsions, especially the heavier salves, *seal off* the surface avenues of escape for the toxins. These poisons then recede or "backtrack", if you will, and blaze a trail to new areas of escape, forming lesions known as satellites. I do not believe it is one particular ingredient that makes the emulsions work. My observations indicate that they will work with any ingredient(s) that can safely seal off the lesions. If this were not so, why is it that circumscribed lesions often disappear equally well after applying substances that are completely foreign to other commodities in their chemical composition that also claim success? It is well known, for instance, that surface tar derivatives are very helpful, but so is castor oil, olive or peanut oil, Vitamin E cream, or—recently being re-investigated, Vitamin D cream. To this list of "sealants" one can even add adhesive tape! The fact is they all work to some degree or another. Some preparations are more pleasant to use than others and have fewer side effects or inconveniences. It is mainly for these reasons that individuals will find one preferable to another.

Gina Cerminara, Ph.D., author and lecturer, in a letter to me some years ago, related the story of a young girl who had psoriatic lesions on her hands. The girl's mother told Dr. Cerminara, who was on a lecture tour at the time, that the daughter, an art student, had accidentally spilled paint thinner on her hands. To her astonishment, the girl later discovered that the lesions had disappeared in the areas saturated by the paint thinner, while in the areas that were not splashed, the lesions remained. I do not know if the lesions eventually returned to the "burned out" areas. The point is that yet another method of sealing off the skin surface was found, although by accident and certainly not a method to be advised, and the psoriatic plaques disappeared.

Why do all of the sealing-off methods have a fair measure of success? I believe it is principally because of the only thing these applications have in common: their ability to act as a barrier to the internal toxins. Again, these toxins have to get out somehow, and until the normal channels of elimination have been opened up, new routes of escape will develop through other areas of the skin. Holding firm to the theory that the toxins are finding their way out through the *sweat glands* infers that the lesions form because of this toxic exodus.

When the patient is treated holistically, all areas and functions of the body are taken into account. Proper elimination of wastes is primary, followed by a diet that is both cleansing as well as nutritious. The external salves and ointments serve as palliative measures. This procedure will cause the toxins to eventually retract and be removed by the now better-functioning excretory system, thus helping to prevent further spreading of the disease.

Physiotherapy—at home

I have often been asked, especially by conscientious patients, if there are any physiotherapy units available that may be used effectively at home. There are indeed, and they can be quite helpful.

The five that I consider most important are:

1. *Whirlpool:* either built in, such as a Jaccuzi bath tub or a portable unit that may be attached to the side of the tub or laid flat in the tub producing air bubbles. Smaller, self-contained units are available for hands and feet.

2. *Steam Bath Cabinet:* for home use. Made of fiberglass with stainless steel and aluminum fittings. The patient sits comfortably in the unit, closes a door but the head is always exposed.

   [Note: The same precautions apply in using a whirlpool or home steam cabinet as they do for taking an Epsom Salt Bath or Professional Steam Bath.]

3. *Electrical Heat Cap, Mitts and Boots:* these are used for treatments of the scalp, hands and feet respectively, in conjunction with various oils.

4. *Humidifier:* Particularly for use in the winter months to offset the dry air caused by artificial heating. A humidifier can be very effective in preventing or alleviating Winter Itch (asteatotic dermatitis). Caution—Units must be thoroughly cleaned out regularly as spores may form that may be inhaled, causing serious respiratory ailments.

5. *Ultraviolet Lamp (optional):* May be used as directed by the patient's dermatologist.

In addition, every psoriatic should have—

a. *A Juicer:* for making fresh vegetable and fruit juices
b. *A Home Enema Device:* especially if constipation is a problem.

The above units are readily available to the general public at a nominal cost. In remote areas where professional services are not available, these home units can be a godsend provided they are used properly and with discretion. They are all a patient needs from a physiotherapeutic point of view. Again, these products become more worthy of consideration when the convenience of using them in the privacy of one's own home is taken into account.

Measures That Have Relieved Itching (A Quick Review)

Since itching is one of the most irritating aspects of psoriasis, I prepared the following summary to give a clear picture of the measures I have suggested:

1. Sodium Bicarbonate Bath
2. Aveeno Bath—to which some patients have added a cup of corn starch.
3. Witch Hazel in Fume Bath (1 tablespoon to 1/2 pint of water)
4. For small areas, direct applications of:
   a. Resinol
   b. Apple Cider Vinegar diluted in water
   c. Olive Oil/Peanut Oil Mixture massage
   d. Witch Hazel, Listerine or Glyco-Thymoline
5. Cool shower or ice cube on small area (not mentioned earlier)

There are a number of prescription as well as nonprescription items available that purport to relieve itching. Whatever works—works! The above nonprescription items are all I ever recommended. Remember, once the internal cleansing process begins to take effect, the annoying itch is the first symptom to disappear and the first sign that the process is working.

No Substitution for Time

There is one basic thing I insist my patients always keep in mind, especially since this regimen is not a "get well quick" procedure. *If I sound redundant it is by intention!*

Psoriasis will not disappear until the basic cause has been removed. Since the basic cause is a buildup of internal toxins over an extended period of time, the removal of these toxins is not an overnight process. The essential requirement in following this regimen is—*give time a chance.* Without it, the effort is worthless. Discipline is an absolute must if results are to be expected and this may not be as rigorous as one might imagine.

One of my patients summed up the attitude needed to apply the psoriasis regimen with complete success in these simple but very wise words:

"It is a discipline only until it becomes a habit—then it takes over!"

Chapter 10

Right Thinking

Albert Schweitzer was once asked the question: "What's wrong with men today?" His answer, sharp and to the point, was: "Men simply don't think!" Of course, not all men fall into that category, but this in itself raises another question. Of those who *do* "think"—what are they thinking about? Are their thoughts of a constructive nature or are they destructive? You see, depending on the nature of their thoughts, their world is built around them. Their bodies and circumstances, whether they want to believe it or not, are the end result of the thoughts they harbor within.

"Of all the beautiful truths pertaining to the soul, none is more gladdening or fruitful of divine promise and confidence than this—that man is the master of thought, the molder of character, and the maker and shaper of condition, environment, and destiny."[1]

So says James Allen in his classic work, *As A Man Thinketh*. Once man realizes that he has, to a great extent, the power to *choose* his thoughts, he would be foolish if he did not decide on a constructive course of thinking. If he then holds to it with faith in the creative power of thought, he will eventually benefit and improve all areas of his life. He is free to choose.

What must he do to realize the healthy life, the good life, the life worth living? He must exercise "right" thinking. Right thinking means choosing a pattern of thoughts designed to benefit him or her without bringing harm to others. Sometimes subtle changes in our thoughts bring about incredible results.

For instance, no one (normally) wants to be sick. But if you say or think the words "I don't want to be sick", you center your thinking on sickness and the chances are you will draw sickness to you. For as you think, so shall you become.

Now, the difference in right thinking is not to say to yourself "I don't want to be sick", but, "I AM HEALTHY!" Here you are making a positive, constructive *present tense* declaration. This affirmation will eventually enter your subconscious mind and manifest in your life if repeated often enough. This will be discussed later in this chapter, "The Mental Formula".

The Wisdom of Thomas Troward

Thomas Troward was one of the world's leading exponents on the power of thought and how it can work to our advantage. He wrote seven books on the subject at the turn of this century. *The Edinburgh Lectures on Mental Science*, perhaps his most popular edition, contains a brief discourse that sums up what he calls the "Train of Causation". To paraphrase: Everything begins with an *emotion or feeling* which gives rise to a *thought*; the *judgement* then decides whether or not to materialize that thought; if the thought is approved by the judgement, the *imagination* is put into motion by visualizing that thought as already accomplished; the *will* then is exercised by holding that picture of the materialized thought until it manifests as a reality in your life.[2]

This train of causation as described by Troward is important to the psoriatics in that they can help the healing process by fixing their thoughts on the idea that their skin is already healed, and visualizing it as an accomplished fact. Patients who follow through on all other measures and add to it this power or visualization have taken a giant step in ridding themselves of this disfiguring disease. The biggest obstacle to overcome is the patient's impatience. Unless he or she is willing to give the process *time* to work, the end result is failure.

Troward emphasizes that once an idea is set in motion by our thoughts, its forward movement cannot and will not stop until the end result is achieved, *unless we ourselves send out opposite, conflicting thoughts that neutralize or nullify our original thought.*

Nothing could be clearer. Or simpler! Nothing begins without a thought setting it in motion. Hold on to the thought, and in ways beyond knowing you will realize it at the appointed time. Do not become confused by trying to intellectualize how it works. This is neither possible nor necessary. And it is open to all humanity. It is, in my opinion, the only explanation for the thought provoking passage that "all men are created equal." It becomes even more understandable to me, however, when I add "once they realize they have the power of thought at their command to set things in motion that work for them."

According to Troward, the very forces of the universe will gather to externalize the thoughts of a single human being. This is why war lords, feudal kings, early church officials and self-proclaimed dictators kept the people subdued either by force or by "Divine" decree. They wanted to prevent the people from *thinking*! The United States of America became the greatest nation on earth in a mere two hundred years (as compared to other nations) because the people had *freedom of thought*.

What has all this to do with psoriasis, one might ask? It has a great deal to do with it when one realizes that we are talking about a *principle*. The principle is *"Thoughts Are Things"*—and you have the power to set in motion the forces that bring all things into being, *including the health of your body!*

Let us put Troward's "train of causation" to practical use and apply the principle to the healing of psoriasis.

The Thought Process

It starts with a feeling or *emotion* to rid oneself of this disease. The *desire* is thereby established. Then, another part of our mental machinery comes into action, the *judgement*, meaning, you must determine whether or not you *truly* want to get rid of this psoriasis. (Some don't, you know.) If, by your judgement, you decide "Yes, I want the psoriasis cured," you have set the goal. Now, how does one attain that goal? By imagining it *as already accomplished* in your mind! This is done by *the will* directing *the imagination*. Simply stated, *the will comes forward and directs the imagination to hold the picture of the desired end result*. This plants a seed, so to speak, in the mental atmosphere which then draws to it progressive building blocks which, in time, continue to grow until, by the law of attraction, the end result is externalized. In this case, it is by the appearance of clear healthy skin.

Now those "progressive building blocks" that coalesce to help bring about the desired end result may be: the knowledge of the regimen to follow, adhering to the diet, practicing internal cleansing, keeping up with the spinal adjustments, never failing to take the teas, etc.

It is most important, however, to understand the relation of the will to the imagination. According to Troward, the function of the will "is to keep the imagination centered in the right direction. We are aiming at *consciously* controlling our mental powers instead of letting them hurry us hither and thither in a purposeless manner, and we must therefore understand the relation of these powers to each other for the production of external results."[3]

Here is something worth memorizing and always keeping in mind: *When the will and the imagination are in conflict with each other, the IMAGINATION ALWAYS WINS!*

In other words, if you cannot *picture* what you desire as accomplished, what you say or even shout over the roof tops is meaningless. More of this is covered later. At this point, it is necessary only to grasp the overall principle; what you visualize through the imagination will, in time, be realized.

To Illustrate

One of the biggest hindrances I have encountered a few times in the healing process is the patient's inner belief that his skin disease must be a punishment from God. With such a belief harbored in the mind, it is next to impossible to obtain positive results. As long as the patient believes he *deserves* to have psoriasis, *he will only succeed in retaining the disease*, for ridding himself of it would, according to his belief, be going against what he thinks is God's will. So even if help is readily available to him, he will avoid it in order to conform to his inner belief.

Fortunately, a young prince of the Medici family in Northern Italy centuries ago did not feel the crippled, deformed body he was born with was the "will of God" and set out to correct it at a very young age by exercising the art of visualization. Because of his physical deformity, he avoided public communication and confined himself to an area within the palace grounds for his studies and meditations. Since he was born a prince, he could have just about anything he wished. What the wise young man ordered would, even by today's standards, be considered eccentric at best and hardly recognized as anything other than wishful thinking.

In the middle of the court where he spent most of his waking hours, he ordered a statue to be carved by a leading sculptor of the day. The statue was to be a classic figure of a powerful Roman centurion; strong, stately, proud, and determined, but with one added factor—the head was to have the likeness of our young prince! Month after month, year after year, the young prince would continue to sit and meditate in his favorite gardens where the statue stood. He would see himself as *he wished he were,* materialized in all his glory every day. With the passing of years, his subconscious mind gradually accepted the message, and the day came when the prince stood straight and strong, a magnificent specimen of manhood, an exact living replica of the model statue.

We learn from this story the power the mind holds over the body and that, in spite of all odds, the seemingly impossible can materialize. We also learn that the key is to *picture* in our mind's eye what we want. In whatever way we help ourselves to picture it is fine, as long as the end result is achieved. We may therefore start our quest for a beautiful clear skin with the happy certainty that God or the Creative Forces are on our side. First we plant the seed, then water and take care of it, then let it grow.

To those afflicted with psoriasis, Edgar Cayce offers help in visualizing the disease gone from their bodies by stating *"There is a cure..."* This completely refutes the age-old, orthodox concept that there is no cure for psoriasis.

This is one important reason why I often have my successful patients meet those just beginning the regimen. It is the most powerful incentive for them to have heart and realize that they can get well. It strengthens their *will* which, in turn, directs the imagination to cling to that picture of perfect health. Then, by the law of attraction, their picture is materialized.

One cannot set a time limit on how long it will take. Each person is a law unto his own being. All I can say with profundity is that by following this method of "right thinking", one's desire is realized in the shortest, natural period of time.

Staying on the "right" road of thinking requires a constant vigil, a "guardian at the gate," if you will, to ward off the intrusion of destructive thoughts or statements or gestures that will distort or even reverse the thought patterns that spell success.

Backfire!

An excellent example of practicing the "guardian at the gate" principle took place right in my reception room.

Two new psoriasis patients met one evening at my office. Both were young ladies with severe cases of psoriasis. I introduced them to each other as I have often arranged for patients to meet in the hope that one would encourage the other. One patient, the positive one, was very enthusiastic at first and quickly began discussing the regimen with the other young lady. It soon became apparent that the other woman did not share her enthusiasm, was filled with doubt, had a defeatist attitude about the entire matter and thought nothing of transferring her discouragement to the patient who was trying to help her.

Later, when I met with the positive patient privately in the treatment room, I was immediately met with: "Dr. Pagano, I appreciate what you are trying to do, but please do not put me in the company of such a person again!" I was confused and rather embarrassed, to say the least, for having patients meet each other usually proves beneficial. Apparently, this situation was an exception. She voiced her dismay at the other woman's attitude and that she did not wish to be mentally "infected" by such thoughts. I explained that my purpose was for "*you* to encourage *her.*" She assured me she tried but soon realized that the other woman was not open to it. In fact, the opposite effect took place. Depression set in on the positive patient, while the other left the office clinging to her negativity.

About six weeks later they met again, purely accidentally, in my reception room. Their conversation seemed to begin where it had ended at their last meeting. The positive patient retained her composure while the other began her negative influence, even though she had shown improvement over the past month. This time, however, right in front of the other patients in the waiting room, the enthusiastic patient cupped her hands over her ears and said strongly and emphatically, "Please, I don't want to hear it!" Nevertheless, the other woman continued her negative remarks. Again, she was met with, "I just told you, I do not want to hear any of your thoughts. Will you please stop!" Finally, when the message got across, the negative person saw she no longer had an audience and backed off.

In the treatment room, the other young lady said, "I'm sorry, Dr. Pagano, but that woman put me in such a depressed state for a month that I refuse to allow her to dump her garbage on me again!" I congratulated her on her forcefulness and determination to guard her mind from thoughts of a destructive nature. She was a perfect example of a person "choosing" her thoughts—selecting them, rather than allowing thoughts from any source to enter her mind. Because she not only refused to allow such an attitude to be absorbed, but also counteracted it forcefully, her whole demeanor was changed. She was more cheerful, smiling, stronger—determined to succeed. And succeed she did. Psoriasis is no longer a problem for her. She was so enthralled by the results that she wrote a lengthy letter to the head of dermatology at one of the country's leading psoriasis research centers, relating her successful experience after years of suffering with the disease.

I did not hear from her for four months. Then a letter came, from which I extract the following pertinent paragraphs:

Dear Dr. Pagano,

It seems like *years* ago that I was plagued with an awful skin disease, that I did absolutely nothing but dwell on, and for which you treated me. With the exception of an occasional outbreak on my face, I am now free of that disease, and will remain on the diet forever. It's hard to believe that not even one year ago I was so depressed about life.

Would you believe that I have not heard a word from that doctor at_____ since I mailed the letter? I'm tempted to send him a copy and ask, "Did you receive this letter?!"

Dr. Pagano, I hope you know how grateful I am for your encouragement and consideration throughout my illness. I would be more than happy to talk to patients of yours who need to hear firsthand how to deal with psoriasis or how I dealt with it. Please don't hesitate to call or write.

Sincerely,

P.A.

It must always be kept in mind that negative influences, of whatever nature, may appear very logical and realistic. At times, there are very strong arguments as to why something should *not* be followed. This is when a patient is to be strongest in his or her resolve. Patients should keep before their mind's eye the successful cases, not the failures, and given time and patience, they will migrate toward a successful result. It may be likened to the man who did not know a thing couldn't be done, so he went ahead and did it! History abounds in true stories of successful outcomes of "impossible" feats. Add your name to the roster of successful outcomes in psoriasis cases and refuse to believe that "there is no cure." There most certainly is one for many people.

"Right Thinking" therefore is practiced successfully once you learn to recognize "Wrong" thinking when it is directed at you. This may not be as easy as it sounds. There are many, often well-meaning individuals, who cast doubts on a patient's efforts. Their thoughts, usually in the form of remarks, can set a patient off track if that patient doesn't learn to recognize them. Subtle remarks such as:

I'll believe it when I see it...
But there's no cure for psoriasis...
Why waste your time...
Here, have another piece of cake...

Identify these remarks for what they are—destructive! My patients know more about the course they are following than do the bystanders. It never fails to amaze me how some people presume to talk authoritatively without so much as reading a book on the subject or attending a lecture. If the patient, by necessity, is living with, or is in the presence of such people constantly, then the best thing to do is follow an age-old philosophy, "Go and tell no man!" Get results first and tell them later. Success requires no explanation—failure permits no alibis.

The Mental Formula of Emile Coué

At first glance it would not surprise me to see a few raised eyebrows when one talks about a mental formula that can help anyone not only in his physical health, but in his outward circumstances, as well. Does such a formula exist? The answer is an unequivocal YES. It was formulated by Emile Coué of France in the mid-19th century. Devoting his life to the study of mental attitude in the healing or alleviation of disease, Coué gained considerable popularity because of his simplistic method of enlisting the aid of intangible healing forces.

Coué reveals a "secret" in which we can use the most powerful instrument in the world, our own mind, to help us. However, first a little should be understood about how our mind functions.

168

In brief, you must look upon your mind as two minds: the *conscious*, the faculty you are using at this very moment reading this book; and the *subconscious*, the faculty of mind that is active when you are asleep or when the conscious faculty is subdued. There is a reciprocal action between the two minds; that is, the conscious mind can (and does) send suggestions to the subconscious mind and, if repeated often enough, the subconscious accepts it as true and brings it forth in your life. The subconscious does not have the power of reason. It accepts as true whatever is impressed upon it. The conscious mind, on the other hand, *does* have the power of reason. It can weigh things and *decide* what it will believe on the basis of the facts placed before it. The subconscious mind then receives these thought projections once the conscious mind is convinced it is the way to go, and accepts it as true and eventually manifests it in your life.

Whether your personal circumstances are of a positive or negative nature, this is the process by which it works. Experiments in modern hypnosis have proven this to be the case time and time again. At present, hypnosis (or perhaps the better term: suggestive therapy) has gained its rightfully deserved, respected place in modern medicine. The most valuable use of hypnosis, however, is the proper use of self-hypnosis. By the understanding and proper application of self-hypnosis, one can decidedly make life easier, fruitful and healthful.

The key to effective self-hypnosis is *repetition*. By constantly repeating a phrase (mentally or verbally) the thought will eventually take hold and begin to manifest in your life. Some people write their desire on little cards and place them in strategic areas where they can view them occasionally. Another very helpful method is to make your own self-hypnosis tape recording and play it each night and every morning. An example of how some of my patients do it may be found in Appendix B.

The first thing that must be dismissed from your mind is the notion that to practice self-hypnosis is to be walking around like a half-dazed zombie! The exact opposite is the truth. You will be more alert and aware. The difference is that your mind will be subconsciously focused on a definite goal, and what the mind is centered on, eventually becomes a reality. Again, it is not necessary for anyone to know the exact intricacies of "how" it works any more than it is necessary to understand the principles of automotive engineering to drive a car. We derive the benefits by learning how to turn the key and direct the power in both instances.

Turning the key toward good health is greatly enhanced when you understand that the thoughts you project into your subconscious mind eventually manifest in your physical body. Although this principle existed since time immemorial, in modern times it was Emile Coué who proved beyond a doubt that truly, you have direct power over the health (and disease) of your body. To some, this may seem to be a rash assumption. It is not. It is a fact of nature, your inherent birthright, your gift of the Divine!

Cognizant of this law then, Emile Coué, after twenty years of experimenting, laid before us a statement, a sentence of a few words that, if practiced daily twenty times a day for twenty days, will enter our subconscious realm and come forth in our life. These most powerful words are:

"EVERY DAY IN EVERY WAY
I AM GETTING BETTER AND BETTER."[4]

Note, it does not indicate improvement in some dim, distant future. It states "I am"—not "I am going to be." It makes clear the time is now, and although you may not be as healthy as you wish to be at the moment—you will become so in the future.

One stipulation, however, is brought out in Coué's works—that is, the affirmation must be within reason. Realistically, there are points of no return when, after abusing oneself with wrong foods, attitudes and emotions for so many years, the problem becomes irreversible. This is also stated in one of the Cayce readings. Even so, this should not deter or discourage a patient, for there are powers of mind that haven't even been tapped. New discoveries are made every day. What has never happened to anyone may happen to you.

To the beneficial formula by Coué, I have added a few phrases that should help the psoriatic in particular.

"EVERY DAY IN EVERY WAY
I AM GETTING BETTER AND BETTER:
THE DIET IS EASY,
NUTRITIOUS AND CLEANSING.
I HAVE NO DESIRE FOR THE FOODS
THAT I KNOW ARE HARMFUL TO ME."

Write it on a small card and keep it at your bedside. These words should be memorized and repeated as often as possible, especially just before you drift off to sleep and as soon as you begin to awaken in the morning, for these are the two periods of time when your subconscious mind is most amenable to suggestion. If, during the night, you find yourself semi-asleep and semi-awake, immediately repeat the suggestion. This period is known as the "muse" and will receive and actually send suggestions of guidance. Coué also recommends you whisper these suggestions so you can hear yourself say them. This is more powerful than just thinking them silently. He also suggested making a string of beads, with twenty nodules on it and repeating the statement twenty times before retiring and twenty times as you awaken. This is but sending desirable thoughts into the realm of your subconscious. It is using the faculty of mind to aid you in the control or even complete alleviation of the disease. It is based on sound, proven, psychological principles and it is yours to use for your betterment.

I can already hear many of my readers say: "Doctor, I tried what you said. I repeated my desires twenty times a day for twenty days and things are not better. In fact, they are worse!" Not an uncommon result. Why? Because as Coué and Troward clearly stated: "When the imagination and the will are in conflict with each other, the *imagination* always wins!" In other words, just to repeat words over and over again is worthless if you cannot see it, feel it, and be it in your imagination. To clearly *picture* it as already part of you is essential for its externalization.

Often it has been said, and with sound reasoning, "Think only of what you want; not of what you don't want!" Why is this advised? I trust my readers now grasp the idea that we draw to ourselves the very thing our minds are centered on.

Thomas Troward in his classic work "The Hidden Power" describes it as follows:

"But people say 'We have not found it so. We are surrounded by all sorts of circumstances that we do not desire.' Yes, you *fear* them, and in so doing you *think* them; and in this way you are constantly exercising this Divine prerogative of creation by Thought, only through ignorance you use it in a wrong direction. Therefore, the Book of Divine Instructions so constantly repeats 'Fear not; doubt not,' because we can divest our Thought of its inherent creative quality, and the only question is whether we shall use it ignorantly to our injury or understandingly to our benefit."[5]

Practicing the Art of Visualization (Alpha and Omega)

We think in pictures, not in words. We use words to describe scenes and from them, we formulate a picture in our mind.

Being deeply engaged in the field of fine art practically all my life, I have learned to visualize scenes completed long before I even place my initial sketch on the canvas. I know in advance where I am going and what I want to accomplish. When the final stroke of the brush is made on the oil painting, it is the materialization of what I *pictured* in my mind and, much to my amazement, often better than I anticipated.

This principle of visualization carries over to every phase of our life and to every accomplishment.

It holds true, most decidedly, in the state of our physical body. A beautiful, well-toned body does not happen by chance. It must first be *desired*; next, *visualized*; then *accomplished*. "Seeing" the end result is the surest way of making it materialize. The means and methods to accomplish this will be doled out to you in stages as you advance. Here's where "stick-to-it-iveness" comes in. Philosophically, it is referred to as the "Alpha and Omega"—the First and the Last. It means the entire series of causation from the first originating movement to the final and completed result.

The *Alpha* is the thought and visualization that the skin can be healed; the *Omega* is the materialization of the end result; the skin is healed. All steps necessary to accomplish the end result (Omega) will be revealed and, if acted upon diligently, cannot miss its mark in time in the vast majority of cases.

Visualizing your skin as pure and clear as you want it to be is not complicated. See it done. The steps will then take place more easily until one day your dream of clear skin will replace the reddened scaly patches of psoriasis. I emphasize to the patient to feel encouraged when little areas of clearing begin to occur, and to disregard the other massive lesions that have not as yet shown any change, for in time, they too will follow suit.

Release from Bondage by Imaging

There is another dimension to the healing process, *imaging*, or the use of mental imagery. Far-reaching, indeed, is the active use of imaging in the regulation of your body, mind and circumstances. Only recently has this concept been recognized and fostered by leading thinkers, although the principle has been in existence since time immemorial.

Dr. Norman Vincent Peale in his "Positive Imaging," informs us of its effectiveness:

> "There is a powerful and mysterious force in human nature that is capable of bringing about dramatic improvement in our lives. It is a kind of mental engineering that works best when supported by strong faith. It's not difficult to practice; anyone can do it. Recently it has caught the attention of doctors, psychologists, and thinkers everywhere, and a new word has been coined to describe it. That word is IMAGING, derived from imagination. An image formed and held tenaciously in the conscious mind will pass presently, by a process of mental osmosis, into the unconscious mind. And when it is accepted firmly in the unconscious, the individual will strongly tend to have it, for then it has you. So powerful is the imaging effect on thought and performance that a long-held visualization of an objective or goal can become determinative. Imaging is positive thinking carried one step further." (Reprinted by permission.)

Dr. William James, the Father of American Psychology, wrote:

> "The greatest discovery of my generation is that human beings, by changing the inner attitude of their minds, can change the outer aspects of their lives...It is too bad that more people will not accept this tremendous discovery and begin living it."

If we are what we are, and where we are, because of the things we image within ourselves, then we can be what we want to be, and where we want to be by the very same law! The difference is we are not *aware* of this fact of life and can use it on a conscious, intelligent level to make our lives what we will. Only now, instead of just wishing, we *imagine* it so—and so it will become.

The Law of Expectancy

The final ingredient necessary to realize your desire is to set the wheels in motion with the underlying sense of *expecting* it to happen. If one doesn't do this, it is like planning a dinner, inviting your friends, preparing the food, buying the right wine, setting the table, dressing to receive your guests—and expecting they will *not* show up!

Does this make sense? Of course not. Having "faith", as I see it, is having the awareness that your thought has creative power by its very nature. It is not something to be attained. *It is!* What is needed is not the power but the knowledge, the awareness that this is a built-in mechanism. It is used every day by everyone. How it is used can be determined by observing the *end result*—for:

> "LIFE'S BATTLES DON'T ALWAYS GO
> TO THE STRONGER OR FASTER MAN—
> FOR SOONER OR LATER, THE FELLOW WHO WINS,
> IS THE FELLOW WHO *THINKS* HE CAN!"

REFERENCES

(Chapter 10—Right Thinking)

1. James Allen, *As A Man Thinketh*, (Mt. Vernon, NY, Peter Pauper Press), p. 9.
2. Thomas Troward, *The Edinburgh Lectures on Mental Science*, (New York, NY, Dodd, Mead & Company, Copyright 1909) p. 85 (By permission).
3. Ibid, p. 84.
4. Emile Coué, *Self Mastery Through Conscious Autosuggestion*, (London WCIA, UNWIN HYMAN LTD., 40 Museum Street)
5. Thomas Troward, *The Hidden Power*, (New York, NY, Dodd, Mead & Company, copyright 1921 by S.A. Troward, 1961 by Dodd, Mead & Company) pp 97-98 (By permission).

Chapter 11

The Crowning Glory

Psoriasis on the Scalp

Psoriasis on the scalp is one of the most unsanitary, uncomfortable, and unpleasant manifestations of the disease which can occur, and the self-consciousness a patient develops, because it is so visible, makes it all the more disturbing. Through the years, I have worked out a hair treatment and shampoo that has proven to be quite effective in ridding the scalp of accumulating scales as well as enhancing the healing of the surface cells. Keeping in mind that the real healing comes from within, my patients' comfort and external appearance was improved by following the treatment outlined at the end of this chapter. In severe cases, where there was a thickening of the scalp and heavy scaling, an electric heat-cap treatment was employed. In the less serious cases, a regular shampoo treatment was helpful and the electric heat-cap treatment was made optional.

At first glance the routine may look bothersome, but I urge my patients to try these treatments as least once or twice. They soon realize that the procedures are quite simple and, once understood, they can breeze through them.

To those patients who insist on using hair dyes and artificial coloring, I can only say—make a choice. You cannot get rid of the psoriasis and the grey hair as well, at least not until the condition clears up. One patient with a severe scalp condition began our conversation with, "Don't tell me not to color my hair. I'll do anything you say, but not that." The fact is, she didn't follow through on any other measures either. Result—she still has her psoriasis as much as ever and is no longer my patient.

The patients *must make a choice*! Which is more important, their vanity or their health? They must decide and act accordingly.

Does Psoriasis Cause Hair Loss?

There is no question in my mind that psoriasis on the scalp can and does cause hair loss particularly if the lesions become too thick. For some patients, hair loss becomes a major concern when they find their hair falling out in "clumps."

When you realize that the hair follicles extend only a fraction of an inch into the subcutaneous cellular tissue of the scalp, it is easy to understand that hair loss is not only possible, but can be expected when psoriasis affects the deeper layers of the skin. This is why the scalp should be shampooed gently, and with the fleshy part of the fingertips rather than the nails.

There is one encouraging note, however, in the majority of cases that I have treated, the hair grew back completely as the internal cleansing process took place.

One of my patients, a college boy with a devastating case of generalized psoriasis, and considerable hair loss, surprised me with a quick visit during his summer vacation to show me how well he was doing. Except for a few minor spots near the lower rib cage and a small area on his back, he was virtually clear of the lesions which at one time had covered most of his body. For a few months he had neglected drinking his saffron tea, but knew that once he resumed drinking it on a regular basis, the problem would rectify itself. I noted that he had trimmed down considerably, looked healthy and strong, and had a crop of hair thick enough to stuff a mattress.

He explained that the regrowth of his hair was one of his greatest joys, for when the disease was at its peak, he had been losing his hair by the handful. The only areas that did not regenerate were those he "picked" at, thus destroying the root of the hair follicle. This is certainly understandable, for if the root is preserved, the shaft of the hair can regenerate completely. He, as well as many others I have treated through the years, was a living example. Therefore, I advise my patients not to despair if psoriasis on the scalp is causing hair loss. It is possible that the hair can come back, in all its glory, healthier and stronger than ever.

Psoriasis Along The Hairline

Two products stand out above all others as having a beneficial effect for psoriasis along the hairline, back of the ears, and in small circumscribed areas on the scalp itself. They are Baker's P&S Liquid and Carbolated Vaseline. Although covered previously in my chapter "External Applications," I feel they deserve being mentioned again. These products may be applied either with fingertips, Q-Tips, or an Orange stick. They are to be rubbed in deeply but with care not to cause damage with fingernails. Remember, the skin is traumatized enough already.

For Itchy Scalp

It may be hard to believe, but common household mouth washes are among the best products readily available to relieve itching of the scalp. They are: Lavoris, Listerine, and Glyco-Thymoline. By rubbing them gently into the scalp in cases of dandruff or scaling, considerable relief can be immediate. These mouth washes can also soothe a scalp that has flared up after an electric heat-cap/oil treatment was applied.

In the case of generalized itch all over the scalp, the mouth washes may be diluted in a quart of warm water and used as a rinse or they may be applied full strength, with the fleshy part of the fingertips, to specific spots that itch.

Another anti-itch remedy used successfully by several of my patients is a mixture of two ounces of apple cider vinegar or white vinegar to six ounces of lukewarm water. It is mixed, then slowly poured over the entire head. It is then rubbed in gently and left on for about one-half to one minute. It is rinsed with lukewarm water, followed by a final rinse of water as cool as is comfortable.

Above all things DO NOT SCRATCH this can only lead to spreading of the psoriatic lesions, bleeding, and possibly infection.

The Shampoo Treatment and an Electric Heat-cap Treatment that I have worked out for my particular patients is detailed as follows:

SHAMPOO TREATMENT FOR A SCALY PSORIATIC SCALP
(As my patients are directed)

Once or twice a week or as deemed necessary

Necessary items:

(a) Large cake of Cuticura soap or Cuticura shampoo (preferred), or Z-Tar shampoo or an olive oil-based shampoo (as alternatives).

(b) Unlined shower cap (or disposables)

(c) One Handi-Wipe, or absorbent cotton strips

(d) One 8 oz. measuring cup

(e) One timer

(f) One bottle of apple cider vinegar (for thick hair), white vinegar (for fine hair), or fresh lemons (alternative).

Notes:

1. Psoriatic patients should never use any form of color or dye on their hair, especially when sores and scales are prevalent on the scalp, as this may very well cause an inflammatory, allergic, or even infectious reaction. Therefore, the following instructions for shampoo treatment should only be applied to the natural scalp.

2. Because of adverse effects on several patients who used a hair dryer or blow dryer, I advise my patients not to use such electrical appliances. It is preferable that their hair be allowed to dry naturally.

Shampoo Treatment:

1. The hair is wet thoroughly with warm water.

2. Lather is made using Cuticura soap (or alternative shampoo). Lather is worked into scalp for a few moments. Water and soap is added as

lather disappears. Plenty of lather is essential while massaging it into the scalp, using tips of fingers. Using nails is to be avoided.

3. The hair is then piled on top of the head. A shower cap, is put on and a handi-wipe is placed around the inside edge under shower cap to prevent liquefying suds from running into the patient's eyes, face, and neck.

4. Timer is set for ten minutes. If the scalp is exceptionally inflamed with sores instead of scales, the time is reduced to five minutes.

5. After the time is up, the hair is thoroughly rinsed with fairly warm *running* water.

6. Steps 1 through 5 are repeated followed by a thorough rinse again. Excess water is squeezed out.

7. Two ounces of apple cider vinegar or white vinegar is poured into a measuring cup. The cup is then filled with six ounces of lukewarm water. It is mixed and slowly poured over the entire head. Scalp must be completely covered. The vinegar solution is very gently massaged into the scalp for about half a minute. (It may sting a little if there is some breakage on the scalp, but it is nothing to worry about.) The solution is left on for two minutes. It is then rinsed with lukewarm water, finishing with water as cool as the patient can comfortably stand.

8. The hair is towel dried and set without using any setting lotions or hair spray.

Note: As an additional aid for sores appearing along the hair line, the use of *carbolated vaseline* is suggested. After completing the above method of shampooing, the fingertips or a Q-Tip is used to apply carbolated vaseline to circumscribed sores that may be in the scalp. The Q-tip is wet first, the water is squeezed out, then the Q-Tip is dipped into the jar of carbolated vaseline and applied gently to the sore areas (not too much). If the Q-Tips prove to be too flexible, an "orange stick" is used. Cotton is rolled on the end, soaked, water is squeezed out and applied the same way. Bakers P&S Liquid or Hydrophilic Ointment may be used as an alternative to Carbolated Vaseline.

If the scalp is very scaly, treatment should be applied twice a week. Patient should see results after approximately ten to fifteen treatments (often sooner). Some see results even after the first application.

ELECTRIC HEAT CAP/OIL TREATMENT

Twice a month
or as deemed necessary

Necessary items:

(a) Electric heating cap (may be obtained at health and beauty aid stores, drug stores or discount stores selling electric appliances)

(b) Olive oil and peanut oil—50/50 mixture

(c) Baby shampoo

(d) Fresh lemons or white vinegar

(e) One 8 oz. measuring cup

Treatment:

1. The scalp is shampooed as described in steps 1 through 5 of Shampoo Treatment. The hair has to be washed only once.

2. After rinsing (step 5), a towel is used to gently pat the hair dry. *The scalp is not to be rubbed.*

3. The scalp is covered with the olive oil/peanut oil mixture (preferably warmed). This is gently rubbed into the scalp using the fingertips, not the nails. The oils are concentrated on the more inflamed areas.

4. An electric heat cap is placed over entire scalp using medium heat for twenty minutes.

5. Heat cap is removed and the oil is washed out with baby shampoo. Again, rubbing the scalp harshly is avoided. In order to remove the oil completely, a second shampoo may be necessary.

6. The hair is rinsed a second time, this time using the juice of one fresh lemon dissolved in eight ounces of warm water. Note, however, that should the hair be dyed or colored, a slight discoloration will take place. As an alternative to using the lemon rinse, a white vinegar rinse is applied consisting of two ounces of vinegar and six ounces of lukewarm water.

7. A final rinse is made with lukewarm *running* water and a towel is used to gently pat the hair dry.

Note: Mouth washes such as Lavoris, Glyco-Thymoline and even Listerine can be beneficial when rubbed *gently* into the scalp in cases of dandruff or scaling, as well as cases of flare-up after an oil treatment. They have also been suggested in the event of severe itching of the scalp.

Chapter 12

Psoriasis on the Hands & Feet

After considerable thought, I concluded that psoriasis on the hands and feet deserved a chapter devoted solely to those portions of the anatomy for two reasons:

1. Psoriasis on the hands and feet has long been recognized as one of the most treatment-resistant forms of the disease.

2. More demands are placed on the hands and feet than on any other part of the human anatomy. To be afflicted with psoriasis on these areas can be more devastating than having it anywhere else on the body, except for the relatively rare instance when it appears on the face. This is true from a visual as well as mechanical point of view regarding the hands, while the effects of weight-bearing make lesions on the feet extremely painful.

Patients with psoriasis on the hands, for instance, are extremely self-conscious and do whatever they can to avoid exposing their hands during business or social engagements. True, psoriasis is not contagious, but how many people know that? Or even care? They look upon it as unsightly and possibly contagious, so the patient feels compelled to keep them hidden as much as possible.

In the case of psoriasis on the feet, even though they are not ordinarily exposed, the awkward, crippling gait the patient assumes is a dead giveaway that all is not right with that person.

The following measures have proved to be very effective for psoriasis of the hands and/or feet with my particular patients:

1. Soak hands or feet in hot epsom salts water, preferably in a whirlpool, for twenty minutes.

2. Pat dry and immediately massage warm peanut oil or a combination of peanut oil and olive oil, well into the hands or lower limbs and feet whatever the case may be. Castor oil can be used in the same way with equal effectiveness.

3. Place a "baggy" over the hands or feet after they have been massaged with the oils and put on white gym socks or eliminate the baggies and use only the gym socks. Leave on for at least 30 minutes or more— better yet, overnight.

On Very Difficult Cases

When the scales are very hard, sharp and crusty on the soles and heels of the feet I have advised the following—the results can be most gratifying: (This procedure may also be used on the palms of the hands which at times can become as coarse as canvas.)

Necessary items: Epsom Salts • Peanut Oil • Sodium Bicarbonate (Baking Soda) • Castor Oil • Baggies (or cotton or disposable latex gloves) • White Gym Socks.

Procedure:

A. Begin with the hot Epsom Salts bathing of the feet or hands preferably in a whirlpool.

B. Next, massage warm Peanut Oil into the hands or feet and lower limbs.

C. After the oil is absorbed, massage a paste-like mixture of Sodium Bicarbonate (Baking Soda) and Castor Oil into the entire area.

D. Place plastic baggies over the feet, then white gym socks, and leave these on for at least one-half hour. (Many patients leave them on overnight.) The same procedure applies to the hands when they are severely affected. In the case of the hands, disposable-type plastic gloves are also readily available and may be used if desired. Remember, the plastic bags may be eliminated in favor of using only the white gym socks for both hands or feet after they have been massaged with the oils. As discussed in my chapter "External Applications," the plastic wrap or rubber gloves may cause an irritation under the skin because of the sweating it causes in both psoriasis and eczema.

Note: If the Epsom Salts Bath and/or the Baking Soda and Castor Oil mixture proves to be too irritating to open sores in the beginning, wash them off in plain, warm water and avoid using this procedure until the cracks and sores heal over. If such is the case, I advise my patients to use only plain warm water in the whirlpool followed by massaging peanut oil or castor oil only (without the baking soda) and cover with the baggy and/or sock. This is to be followed until the underlying sores and cracks are healed over.

When Washing Dishes

In the case of dish washing, it is best to use the rubber gloves. When psoriatic or eczema skin comes in contact with laundry or dish washing detergent the result can be an irritated, fiery reaction to the hands. Sometimes the rubber gloves cause this irritation even if they are on for only a few minutes. If this occurs, cotton gloves should be worn first, followed by the rubber gloves.

Two Stories of Success

Two of the most severe cases of psoriasis on the hands and feet that I have ever encountered are those of Mr. S.R. (see color photo section) and Mrs. B.K. (see photos in this chapter).

In the case of S.R., we have a fine young man who had suffered with this problem for seventeen of his nineteen years. Throughout his life no expense was spared by his devoted parents in their search for effective remedies. None were found. All of his much-loved sports activities were curtailed or became impossible to perform. His social life was always under a cloud. He would avoid shaking hands with male friends, and rarely attempted to hold a girl's hand. It took four to six months, but S.R.'s hands and feet became as smooth as silk, with not a lesion or an abrasion to be found on them. He followed instructions to the letter, and in June 1985 he was able to tell his encouraging story at a lecture I delivered at Virginia Beach. In a videotape made that day, entitled "Project: Psoriasis", S.R. appears along with four other patients of mine from the New York area before a standing-room only audience to tell how his recovery took place.

He made it very clear that diet appeared to be the culprit in his particular case. Tomatoes, he discovered, played havoc with his hands and feet. Since he had psoriasis only on these areas of the body, he made a concerted effort to get relief from the external effects of the condition.

Adhering strictly to the recommendations, he would first soak his feet (or hands) in an Oster Whirlpool massager. I recommend this unit above all others as it has several cycles and keeps the water quite warm. It is a most valuable investment for a patient with this problem. After about fifteen or twenty minutes of soaking in the hot whirlpool, S.R. would pat his feet dry and while they were still warm and even red from the treatment, he would saturate all the affected areas with the olive oil/peanut oil mixture or castor oil, and massage it deeply into the skin. After a few minutes of this massaging, being very generous with the oils, he would place a large plastic bag over each foot, followed by a clean white gym sock, and retire for the night. In the morning, he would remove the socks and bags, wash his feet thoroughly and then dress according to his plan for the day and go about his business. Sometimes he would apply a light coating of castor oil on his feet, cover them again with plastic bags and gym socks and leave these on even at work.

His remarkable recovery, with complete regeneration of the surface epithelium of both feet, is vividly shown in the color photographic section (case of S.R.). His hands cleared up simultaneously with his feet by means of the same procedure. His story, among others, is an inspiration to all psoriatics.

Another case of remarkably quick and complete healing was that of B.K. (see black and white photographs in this chapter). Her psoriasis was all over the body, but most severe on the soles and heels of her feet. It was so painful that she had to have friends support her under the arms in order for her to walk into my office. In cases as severe as this, as previously described, it called for saturating the feet with a poultice of castor oil and baking soda after the initial soaking. This method of treatment was continued until all areas softened, and then only pure castor oil or the olive oil/peanut oil mixture was used. "Baggies" and socks were placed over the feet every night, and areas that had been covered with razor sharp scales became smooth and clear in a few months. Several years passed before I decided to inquire of my patient as to how she was doing. Her answer was "No problem!" When and if she has a "flare-up" she knows exactly why she does, places herself back on the regimen and the slight recurrence disappears. In other words, her life is in order and has been ever since her initial clearing. In her case, the dietary culprits proved to be tomatoes, shellfish and vinegar.

A LASTING RESULT:

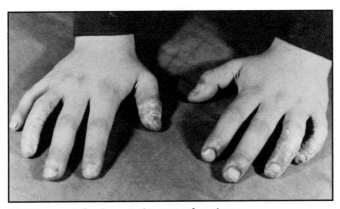

(A.) Young A.S., Age: 5, At start of regimen.

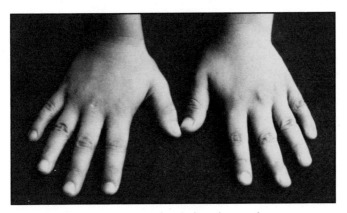

(B.) Nine months later—patient's hands are clear.
Sixteen years later (1991), at age 21, his hands remain clear.

HOME WHIRLPOOL THERAPY FOR HANDS OR FEET
—Oster Unit—

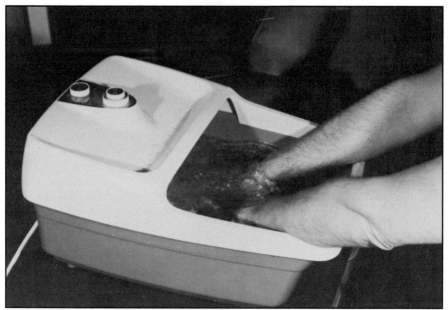

Fig. 12-1   Hands: (Whirlpool treatment)

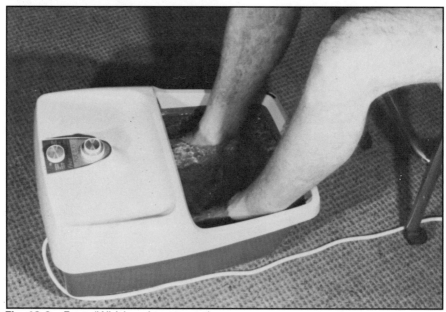

Fig. 12-2   Feet: (Whirlpool treatment)

Patient: B.K.
Afflicted: 2 years

This patient could not even have bed sheets touch her skin.
(See also Chapter 2 "Does It Work?" Patient B.K.)

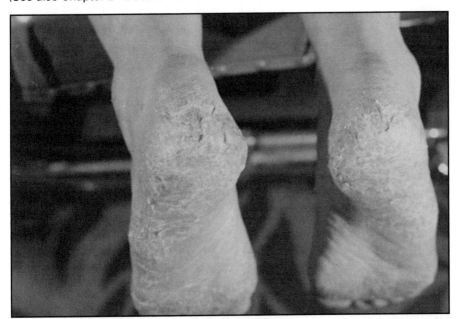

Fig. 12-3 Above photo taken at start of regimen.

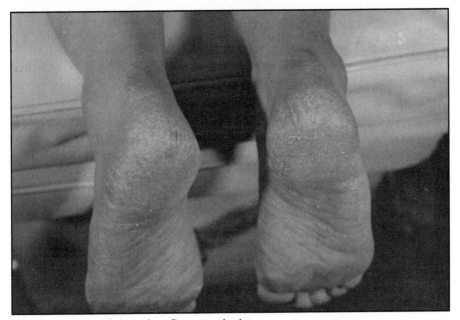

Fig. 12-4 Above photo taken five months later.
Eleven years later, the patient remains in control of the disease. 191

Patient: L.M.
Afflicted: 14 years

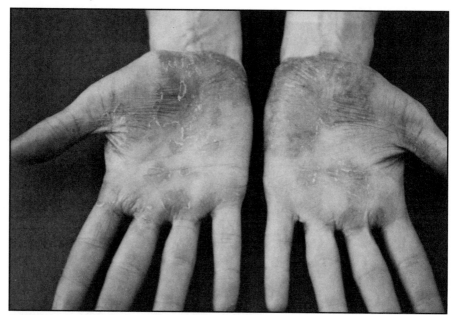

Fig. 12-5 Above photo taken at start of regimen.

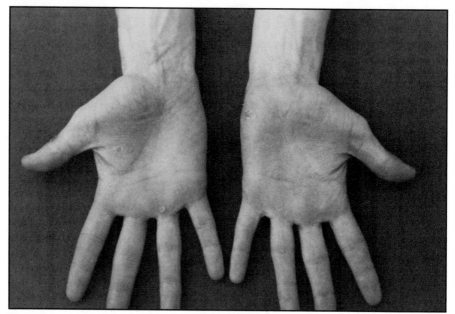

Fig. 12-6 Above photo taken fourteen months later.

A Word of Caution

Once clearing of the hands, especially the palms, has taken place, the patient must not make the mistake of abusing them through rough manual activity. Remember, the surface cells are new. The deeper layer, the dermis, is just beginning to come back to life. These areas need time to fully recuperate from the ordeal they have been through perhaps for many years.

One successful patient was so pleased with the results obtained in the palms of his hands, after suffering with it for twenty years, that he thought he could go out and chop wood. He did this for several hours. It took a few days, but the effect of that activity threw him into a spin for his hands flared up to a marked degree. He thought he was having a relapse. It was nothing of the kind. I explained to him that it was a natural reaction to the localized abuse of his hands. Another patient, after clearing, began working with solvents, gasoline, etc. without wearing protective gloves. A similar reaction occurred, for the same reason -"too much too soon." I advised them to curtail such activity and realize that for about six months after healing, the hands may be used in a normal manner but never to the point of becoming traumatized. This is why I emphasize using protective gloves even when washing dishes. The detergents could play havoc with the hands. Traumatizing the feet also takes place if the patient plays basketball or tennis too soon for reasons previously stated. In other words, be gentle to your hands and feet they will love you for it.

Summary

All other things being equal that is, diet, spinal adjustments, enemas, etc. the best external treatment for patients with psoriasis on the hands and feet was hot soaks in epsom salts water or home whirlpool for about fifteen to twenty minutes, followed by thorough massages with peanut oil, castor oil or an olive oil/peanut oil mixture applied deeply into the hands or from the knees down in the case of the feet. At times, plastic bags were placed over the area treated followed by a white gym sock and left on for at least thirty minutes, often overnight. Lately, however, I am recommending gym socks be used directly over the oils rather than using plastic bags. This measure not only stops irritation but also prevents "skin-rot," which may possibly occur with those patients who are severely afflicted.

At first these measures were carried out every night. After improvement took place, treatment was cut back to three times per week, then once a week, and eventually eliminated altogether. On occasions when the castor oil/baking soda poultice was too caustic and gave a burning sensation, it was temporarily halted in favor of plain castor oil.

In cases of psoriatic arthritis, the hands and feet are usually affected. The same treatment has proved equally beneficial in the vast majority of these cases, but, invariably more time is needed.

A Lesson in Patience

An example of how patience eventually pays off is provided by one of my male patients, who had psoriasis only on the palms of his hands. (See Patient: L.M., this chapter.) After suffering for fourteen years and being treated extensively by orthodox procedures without results, Larry M. came to me as a last resort. In his case, it took fourteen months to clear his palms totally. This may seem like a long time to some, but he feels it was a small price to pay for a lifetime of freedom. "Fourteen months after being afflicted fourteen years isn't bad" according to Larry. After he cleared, I did not see him in my office again for five years. When he returned in 1985, it was for a back problem, his hands were still completely clear, even though he now "cheats" somewhat on his diet. He too, appears in my video production.

Even though the procedures in this chapter dealt primarily with external applications, diet still was the chief culprit in every case. It is interesting to mention that another patient of mine who suffered with psoriasis on the palms of his hands was practically addicted to cajun (blackened) foods. He was improving quite nicely when on the prescribed diet, but one day while dining out the food he ordered was served cajun style, which as most people know is prepared with hot spices. He was about to send it back but decided to try it anyway since he hadn't had it in such a long time. Enjoy it he did but to his dismay, the palms of his hands reacted almost immediately. He felt the "sting" in them within a few hours, convincing him that the hot spices somehow did indeed find their way to the palms of his hands.

What is the common denominator, in the cases presented in this chapter, of people who cleared up their psoriasis by following this alternate route when all else failed? Patience and Persistence! In each of these cases, the patient fully recognized that he or she had exhausted all available therapies. In desperation, they followed the course I offered them. Each was healed to their satisfaction with everlasting joy and gratitude. Today, they are among my most helpful patients in convincing others to follow through with the regimen and to have faith. They are living examples of success achieved by believing that when you do the right thing, the right result will follow.

Chapter 13

The Healing Process

In an earlier chapter I mentioned the fact that one of my biggest problems in caring for psoriasis patients is holding their confidence until they see visible signs of true healing. Once this occurs the patient is convinced that the process is working and that he/she is not wasting time and will usually follow through with greater enthusiasm.

Less itching, less scaling, and a general feeling of well being, if you remember, are the first indications that the procedure is taking effect. There are, however, visible signs that follow that act as proof-positive indications of healing that all psoriasis patients should learn to recognize. I look upon them as *types* of healing that manifests in one of the following ways:

1. Healing becomes apparent from the start and continues to a successful outcome without drastic changes in the skin other than a slow, but steady, gradual fading away of the lesions.

2. In circumscribed lesions, new skin begins to break through at the center of the lesion, giving a bulls-eye effect, and spreads to the outer edges (periphery) of the lesion, forming a "rim", which in time also fades away. This type of clearing is observed best in the common vulgaris form of psoriasis.

3. The existing lesions spread out, join other lesions (coalesce) and appear as massive sheets of inflamed skin. The difference is the diseased areas are now notably thinner, less scaly and gradually get lighter and lighter. New, regenerated skin begins to appear as a

"spotty" effect which ever widens until the inflamed areas disappear leaving the patient with a new skin surface. It is this latter type of healing that we will primarily deal with in this chapter.

When I am sure the patient followed the regimen faithfully and such drastic changes occur as described in #3, I conclude without reservation that they are truly on the road to recovery. It is only a matter of time before the apparent spreading flare-up will subside for that type of reaction is part of the healing mechanism in that particular case. When the new skin breaks through, and continues until all inflamed areas disappear, the joy of accomplishment on the part of the patient as well as the physician, is indescribable.

A Very Special Case

Early in June of 1990, the father of a beautiful little girl, age 7, called in a state of total desperation. His little daughter, L , developed a case of psoriasis over the past year. She had been diagnosed and treated by three dermatologists during this time without satisfactory results. Upon consulting with medical specialists at a leading psoriasis center in New York City, he was informed that his daughter would have it all her life. Their recommendation was treatments with ultraviolet light several times a week, which would be administered at the hospital, as well as the application of cortisone creams. They left the hospital with a sense of futility. "This is it!" they pondered. For the rest of their daughter's life, they would have to fight this terrible disease.

It was the day after they left the hospital that they heard of me and my work, and called immediately for a consultation. A more loving family is not to be found. Their devotion and concern for each other struck me as the stuff dreams are made of.

We felt an instant rapport with one another. When I showed them the results I had obtained on a number of similar cases, their attitude instantly changed from total despair to possible hope. They all agreed to follow the regimen, especially the diet, and help little L in any way they could.

At first her skin seemed to react violently, then, like magic, the psoriasis simply disappeared. It took a little over three months for L to clear with only the slightest spot or two on her scalp remaining. Even these minor areas continued to fade with time. Her story is best told in the following photographic sequence:

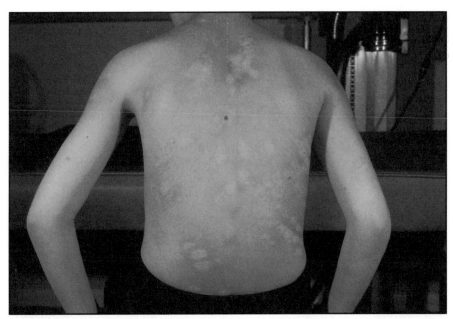

Fig. 13-1
Taken 6/15/90 at Start of Regimen. Lesions are thick and scaly.

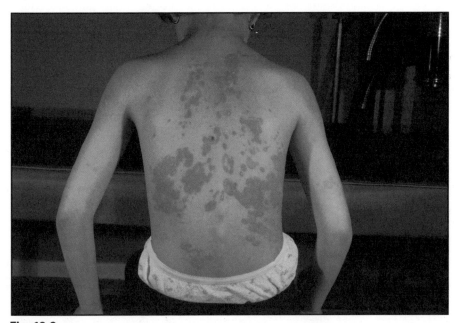

Fig. 13-2
Taken 6/26/90 (after 11 days)—a generalized flare-up occurs.

199

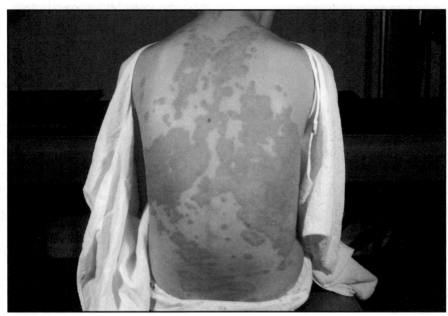

Fig. 13-3
Taken 7/13/90 (after 28 days)—the lesions coalesce and become widespread, but there is less scaling and the lesions are thinner with signs of new skin appearing.

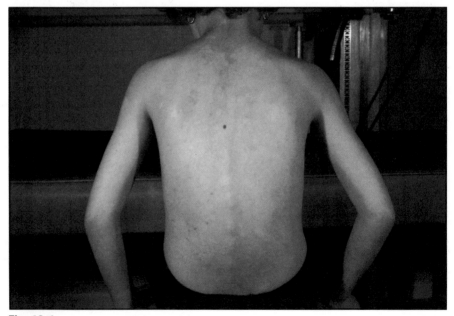

Fig. 13-4
Taken 8/30/90 (after 48 days)—new skin replaces all inflamed areas with only the slightest remains of previous lesions.

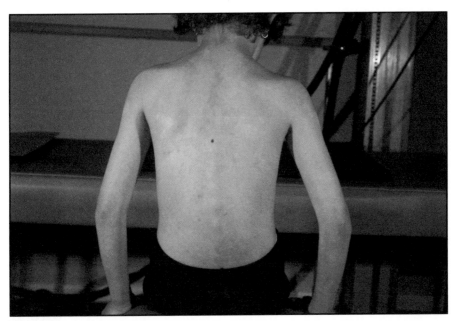

Fig. 13-5
Taken 9/24/90 (after 73 days)—all lesions disappear. Entire torso is regenerated.
Total healing time: 3 months, 1 week.

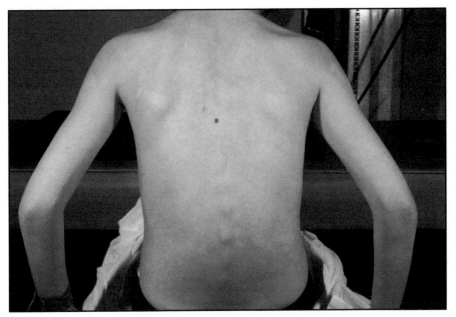

Fig. 13-6
Taken 10/26/90 (one month later)—a close-up view. Patient remains clear.

This particular case stands out in my mind as one of the most profound because I *know* she did not deviate whatsoever from the regimen. Her devoted parents kept in touch with me constantly, assuring me that she did not, would not, stray from the regimen. As has happened with other cases in the past, when an initial flare-up took place (Fig. 13-2) and began to spread, coming together into solid sheets, (Fig. 13-3), her parents became most concerned. It seemed everything was taking a turn for the worse. Drawing on past experience, my only advice was, "Keep going! Do not stop what you are doing." They agonized, but reluctantly agreed. Soon the turning point came; new skin began to appear and shortly thereafter the lesions faded away (Fig. 13-4). The little girl's grateful father called to say "It's just amazing, I can't believe it, the lesions are all gone!" (Fig. 13-5). A follow up photo was taken one month later. The patient remains clear (Fig. 13-6).

In the past, when such a reaction took place with some patients, they would quickly resort to orthodox methods to try to calm the skin down. I can understand this, but in so doing they thwart the process and render this particular research invalid. In the case of this little girl, however, it was the first time I ever had the opportunity to film the sequence without disruption or deviation of the regimen. Such a photographic progression has never been done before and should encourage others to continue with the procedure knowing they are on the right track even when major flare-ups occur. Contrary to the assumption that the disease is running rampant and getting out of hand, despite appearances, *it is a sign that the process is working.*

Incidentally, the biggest dietary violation that I determined contributed to this girl developing psoriasis was tomato ketchup! Her mother informed me that she spread tomato ketchup on bread practically every day for years. Once this practice stopped, combined with all other suggestions, the internal healing process began and continued to a successful conclusion.

Most important of all is the fact that this little girl was relieved of psoriasis at an early age thereby warding off what very well could have been a lifetime of illness, discouragement, disfiguration and untold expense on the part of her parents. True, she probably will always have to be aware of her diet, but with such knowledge she will also experience the greatest joy of all—*that of never having to fear the disease again.*

Throughout my lifetime I can honestly say that I have received, in one way or another, a fair share of awards and citations honoring something I may have accomplished. As I look back upon those accolades, none can compare with the gift given to me by this little girl. "She just wanted to do something special for you" is how her mother described her appreciation. Below is reproduced a personally handdrawn color illustration of her sentiments. I consider this a work of art that will always have an honored place in my office and home as a reminder, that in spite of all professional advice to the contrary, one need not live with this disease.

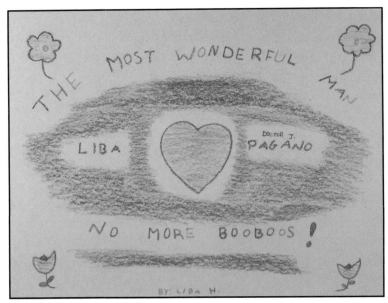

Fig. 13-7 A Special Gift

Chapter 14

Pushing the Panic Button

Crises arising out of following this regimen have been few and far between. In the past ten years or more, I cannot think of a single case where something occurred that put us in a spin. From experience, I've learned to alert my patients to certain changes, even if they are minor, that may occur while on the regimen, particularly in the first weeks. This warning usually takes care of any undue alarm and the patient continues to follow through without concern.

There are, however, two reactions in particular that understandably disturb some patients regardless of my pre-warnings.

1. *New* lesions may pop out in different areas and it may appear that the disease is spreading. (Such as the case of little L as depicted in the previous chapter)

2. A weight loss (sometimes considerable) may occur, but is usually desirable.

These two, if they occur, are the most troublesome to deal with.

My advice is: (1) Ignore the new lesions and carry on with the regimen. In every case to date, the new lesions eventually faded and disappeared. (2) In the case of weight loss (if it bothers them) I advise my patients to "double up" on the food they are permitted to consume but not to go overboard. Hunger should never be a problem, but remember, even eating too much of the permitted foods can cause an overtaxation of the digestive process. Moderation is still the keynote. Most patients are overweight anyway because of their former dietary habits.

Family Reactions

A family member's reaction can be as troublesome as a patient's. If, for instance, their child or spouse is not responding one hundred percent from the very beginning, they overreact, discourage the patient and irritate me.

One young patient, rather severely afflicted with psoriasis, followed all instructions in taking his epsom salts bath. Immediately upon completion of the bath, while the pores of his skin were naturally wide open, he covered himself with Cuticura Ointment. This was *not* when Cuticura Ointment was supposed to be used. His body became inflamed. His mother, in a panic, called me and demanded an explanation. What should she do? He was "burning up." After the terror subsided and the accusations ceased, I was able to explain to her what the boy had done. Instead of using the olive oil/peanut oil combination which is called for after an epsom salt bath, he had used Cuticura Ointment all over his body. Obviously, his skin reacted violently. The remedy was simple. Shower away the ointment from the skin. He did, and was relieved immediately. Here was a clear case of familial overreaction, but certainly understandable.

This does not imply that all families will react emotionally. In some instances the parents have been more understanding than me.

As you will recall, one of my youngest patients in the early years of my experimentation was A.S. At the time, I had no explanation why new lesions were forming where they had never been before. Both parent and patient had followed the rules of the regimen religiously. "That's all right, Dr. Pagano," his mother said. "We said we would give you three months and we will stick to it." Stick to it they did. In time, not only the old, but the new lesions had faded away. As A.S.'s mother states, one day they looked and the lesions were simply not there.

From this early experience, I learned and taught my patients to follow through with the regimen without being in a hurry. You cannot set a time limit on the disappearance of the lesions. Those patients that were successful simply did what was required of them without fuss or bother and allowed nature to take its course.

206

When Prompt Attention Is Necessary

Two young, attractive women, who had suffered with psoriasis for many years, began therapy at the same time. They were eager to see the process in action. One even began to show signs of improvement within the first week, especially behind her ears. The other did not show any appreciable change but there was a marked improvement in her eliminations.

After the third week, however, their enthusiasm changed to discouragement. The girl who was so pleased with the healing behind her ears was deeply upset because lesions now broke out all over her face, particularly her forehead. It looked very much like prickly heat but, of course, it was not. The other girl was distressed due to inflamed areas in her genital region. Pruritus (itching) became unbearable, keeping her up all hours of the night. Nothing seemed to help. She reported she was doing well on the diet and other measures if only it were not for the itching.

For the patient with new lesions on her face I advised her to brew a pot of Saffron tea, place a towel over her head and the teapot and allow the tea's gentle vapors (not too hot) to suffuse her face. After repeating this treatment over two days, the lesions began to disappear. By the following week, they were practically gone and her eagerness to continue treatment was renewed.

For the other young lady, I recommended a sitz bath with about one-third to one-half bottle of Glyco-Thymoline mixed in the water. This gave her the first sense of relief in weeks. Later she had only to pat Glyco-Thymoline, full strength, on severely affected areas and the relief was almost immediate.

In both cases, as in others, it was important that quick adjustments in treatment be made before the patient lost faith in the procedure.

Allergic Reactions

Anyone can develop an allergy. It is very important that the patient's allergy history be established before any treatment is undertaken. Allergic reactions can occur from a blade of grass to a strand of hair, not solely from foods or medications. Usually, one's allergic reactions are established *after* they have taken place. Even allergy testing beforehand is not foolproof nor is it completely accurate in its evaluation.

The rule regarding allergies is simple: Once an allergen has been determined, it is best to *stay away from it.*

One out of every ten people in the United States suffers from some major form of allergy. One out of every two may, at some time, experience a minor one. Some allergies have emotional or psychological origins, a great percentage carrying a long family history. The word "allergy" is often used to connote an adverse reaction, due to a mysterious cause.

Physical reactions manifest in a number of ways; skin rash, for one, swelling and irritation of mucous membranes for another. Asthmatic attacks as well as changes in mood or mentality, such as violence, aggression and confusion, can also be attributed to allergens. Reactions can vary from a minor annoyance to incapacitation requiring hospitalization. Regardless of the degree experienced, allergy of any kind should not be taken lightly and whatever measures necessary should be taken to counteract or avoid having them altogether.

A dear friend and patient of mine cannot have the smallest piece of a pecan. If she does, even if it is hidden in a piece of cake, her reaction is severe. It could mean a matter of life or death. Her throat constricts cutting off her air passage. Hospitalization and adrenaline shots are necessary to counteract the allergic reaction. Similar incidents are commonplace with some persons when they consume shellfish. The list of allergens is endless when *all* people are considered. In these cases "pushing the panic button" is *justified.*

The dietary measures outlined in this book for psoriasis, although rare, do, at times, cause allergic reactions in some people. The individual must take the responsibility of determining which ones they are.

For instance, broccoli is a highly desirable vegetable and encouraged as part of the diet; yet, one of my patients has a severe digestive disturbance and skin flareup when she consumes the smallest amount of it. Carrots are to be eaten as often as possible, perhaps as frequently as lettuce and celery. However, if you will recall, I had one patient who could *eat* them without experiencing any problems as long as she did not *touch* them. Upon touching them her fingers would become inflamed immediately and react violently. Another patient cannot even bring a raw apple to her mouth. If she does, her lips swell up like balloons. These reactions, although relatively rare, must be recognized and respected. If a patient finds they are supersensitive to any of the measures called for in this regimen again my advice is clear: *Avoid them!*

Substitutes can always be found for practically every measure. With a little time, patience and observation, one can reach a workable alternative that will help avoid future undesirable episodes.

Color Photographic Portfolio

The following photographic account represents
a cross section of some classic types of
psoriasis cases treated successfully by following the
Cayce/Pagano Natural Alternative approach to the disease.
These patients followed through with *patience
and persistence* bringing about the desired end result.

Permission to use the photographs in this publication has
been granted by each patient. Initials only are used to
protect the patient's right to privacy.

CASE HISTORY

Patient: L.G. (Female)   **Age**: 34   **Afflicted**: 22 years

Diagnosis: Psoriasis (Generalized)—Over 80% of her body was covered.

Previous Management: Extensive orthodox medical procedures for as long as she has had the disease.

Began The Natural Alternative Regimen on: 2/17/83

Results: Within 3 months there was a marked improvement throughout her entire body. This progressive healing continued for the next two years. After clearing to her satisfaction, she remains in control of her condition.

Remarks: The basic regimen, combined with home enemas, played the major role in obtaining these results. This patient also admits that if she stopped smoking, she would have achieved results more rapidly.

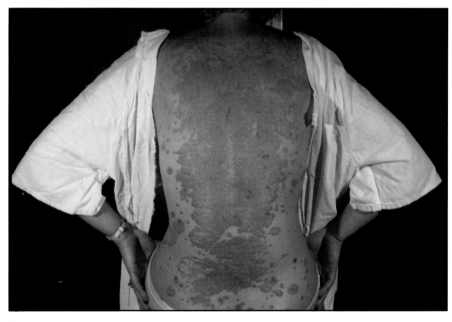

1. Patient before beginning Alternative Regimen—2/17/83

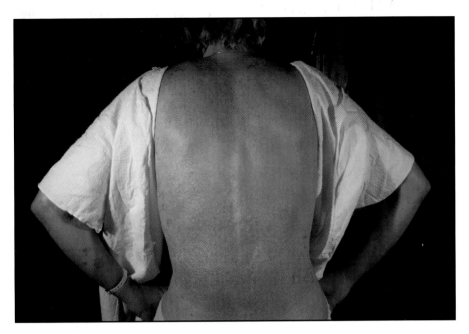

2. Three months later—5/19/83

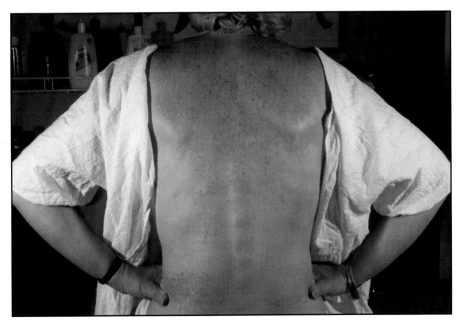

3. Two years later—6/5/85

CASE HISTORY

Patient: J.C. (Male) **Age**: 30 **Afflicted**: 1 year

Diagnosis: Psoriasis (Common/Pustular)

Previous Management: Several medical procedures

Began The Natural Alternative Regimen on: 4/6/84

Results: Marked change in all lesions in 2 months; practically 100% clear in 5 months.

Remarks: This patient remained clear of all lesions for four years despite breaking his diet at times. When lesions began to reappear, he immediately went back on the regimen and brought it under control. Presently (1990) he is no longer plagued with the disease but he must maintain a vigil over his diet and eliminations.

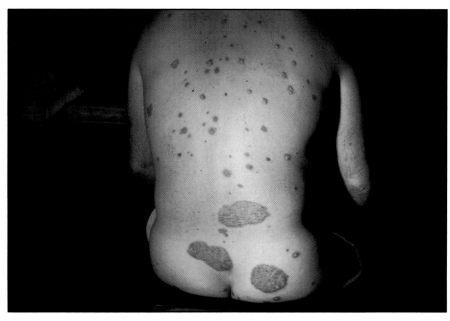

1. Patient before beginning Alternative Regimen—4/6/84

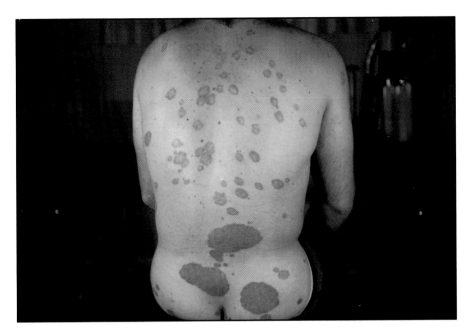

2. Two months later—6/15/84

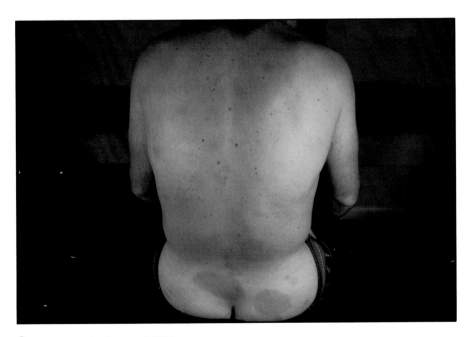

3. Five months later—9/5/84

CASE HISTORY

Patient: J.R. (Male) **Age**: 36 **Afflicted**: 2 years

Diagnosis: Psoriasis (Common Vulgaris)

Previous Management: Under medical care—but not very extensive.

Began The Natural Alternative Regimen on: 7/7/83

Results: Within 4 months the lesions markedly improved. The patient was free of all lesions 6 months after starting the Regimen but then reverted to his old dietary habits and a lesion began to appear again on his left wrist. He learned that dietary control is most important.

Remarks: This patient was extremely overweight at the start of treatment. Within the year that it took to clear his psoriasis, he lost a total of 60 lbs. His figure transformed from total obesity to that of an athlete.

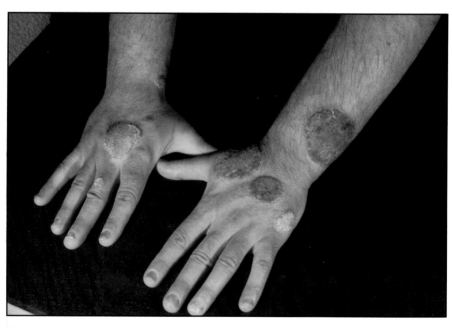

1. Patient before beginning Alternative Regimen—7/7/83

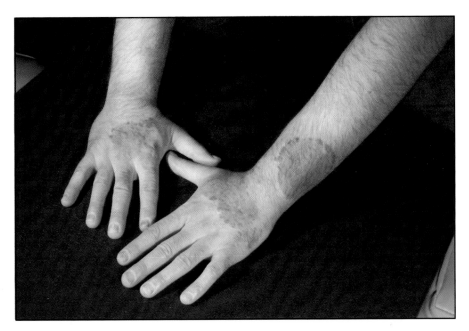

2. Four months later—11/10/83—Lesions visibly fading

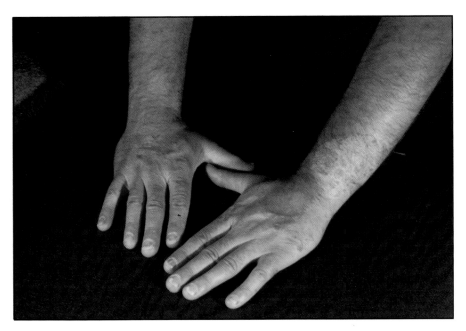

3. Thirteen months later—8/27/84

CASE HISTORY

Patient: S.R. (Male)   **Age**: 22   **Afflicted**: 18 years

Diagnosis: Psoriasis (Pustular)

Previous Management: Extensive orthodox procedures for 18 years.

Began The Natural Alternative Regimen on: 6/10/80

Results: Soles of feet and palms of hands were clear in 10 months. They remain clear 5 years later. Presently (1990) he is in complete control.

Remarks: Only a strong determination to succeed accounts for this young man's success. Now, if there is a slight recurrence, he immediately reverts back to the regimen bringing it under control. As severe as it was, this patient no longer has a problem with psoriasis.

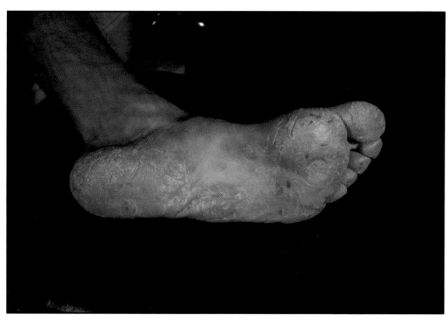

1. Patient before beginning Alternative Regimen—6/10/80

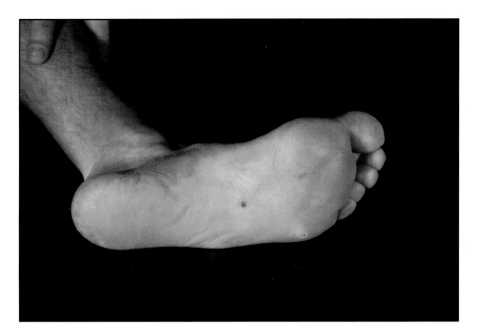

2. Ten months later—4/18/81

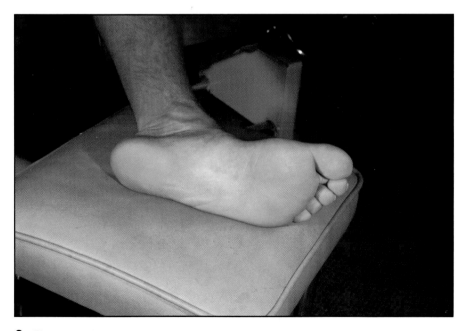

3. Five years later—2/12/85

CASE HISTORY

Patient: A.M. (Female) **Age**: 22 **Afflicted**: 6 years

Diagnosis: Psoriasis (Generalized/Erythrodermic)—Over 90% of her body covered

Previous Management: Extensive orthodox medical procedures—including hospitalization

Began The Natural Alternative Regimen on: 4/2/87

Results: Marked improvement in 1 month; almost 100% clear 3 months later—7/21/87.

Remarks: Diet played a most significant role in healing this patient. Prior to her beginning the regimen, her diet consisted of Pizza and Chocolate practically every day.

Note: In this type of psoriasis, there is an overall redness of the skin surface—not unlike a boiled lobster. The only areas unaffected were the tips of the elbows.

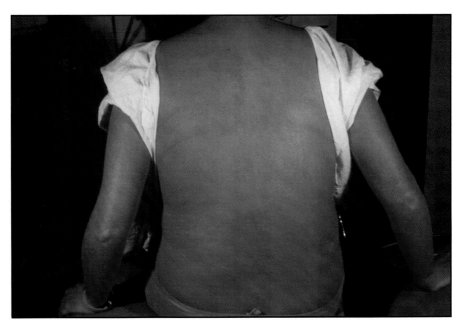

1. Patient before beginning Alternative Regimen—4/2/87

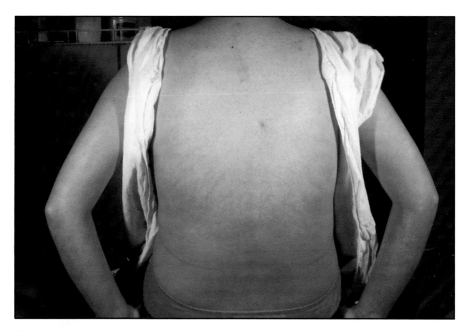

2. One month later—5/5/87

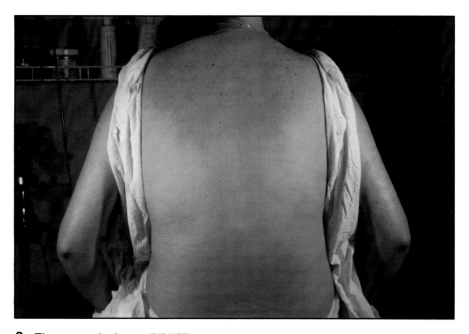

3. Three months later—7/21/87

CASE HISTORY

Patient: M.F. (Female)   **Age**: 22   **Afflicted**: 10 Months

Diagnosis: Psoriasis (Guttate)

Previous Management: Patient had been under the care of three dermatologists before beginning this regimen.

Began The Natural Alternative Regimen on: 3/1/86

Results: The patient was completely clear of all lesions by 7/11/86 (4 months after beginning).

Remarks: At first, results were slow. Rapid healing took place after the patient spent one week at A.R.E. for concentrated hydrotherapy and physiotherapy. In 1990 signs of recurrence began to appear due to straying from the diet for too long a period of time. Once back on the regimen, she again brought the condition under control.

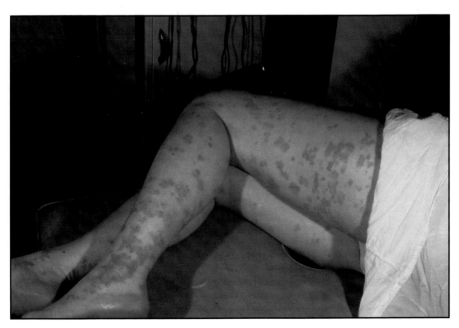

1. Patient before beginning Alternative Regimen—3/1/86

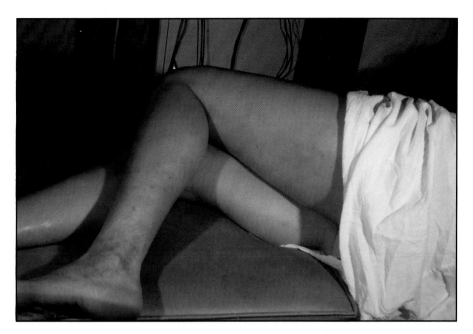

2. Two months later—5/20/86

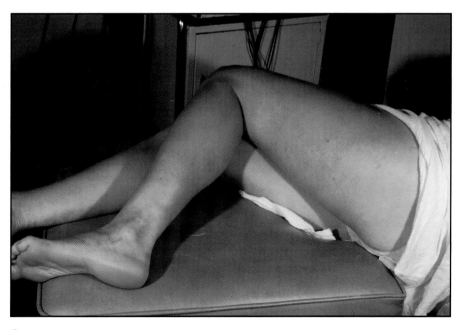

3. Four months later—7/11/86—Clear of all lesions

CASE HISTORY

Patient: T.O. (Female)   **Age**: 14   **Afflicted**: 5 years

Patient: Psoriasis (Generalized)—Over 75% of her body surface was covered with lesions

Previous Management: Various orthodox medical procedures

Began The Natural Alternative Regimen on: 2/23/90

Results: Vast improvement in 2 months.

Remarks: This young girl was successful in her first attempt to follow this regimen in 1987. She had remained clear for over two years before lesions began to appear again and quickly spread through her entire skin surface. It was determined that the reason for the violent outbreak was her straying from the diet for too long a period of time by eating teenage "junk" food and by eating too much of her favorite food—macaroni and cheese! Once she reverted back to the dietary rules of the regimen, spinal adjustments, proper eliminations and the external application of hydrophilic ointment, her skin quickly responded. In two months she was virtually clear of all lesions. She is in complete control of her condition.

Note: This Patient healed so quickly that there was simply no time to take a photo of her at the mid-healing stage; therefore, the only pictures shown are those of the initial stage, followed by the completed, healing stage of her abdomen and back.

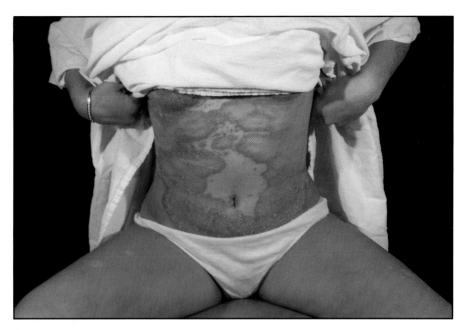

1. Patient before beginning Alternative Regimen—2/23/90

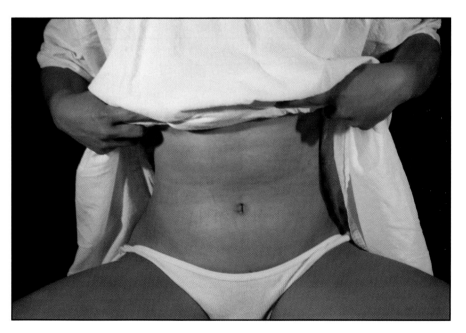

2. Two months later—4/28/90

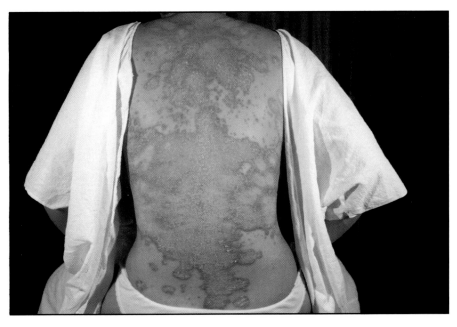

3. Patient before beginning Alternative Regimen—2/23/90

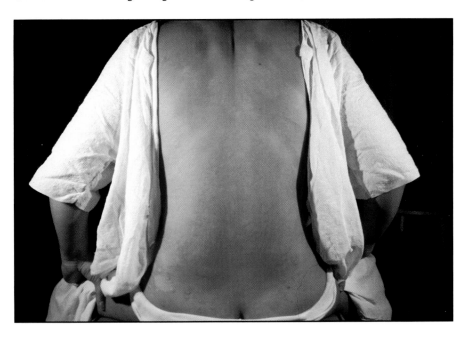

4. Two months later—4/28/90

Chapter 15

The Arthritic Connection
(Psoriatic Arthritis)

Among the millions of psoriatics, a small but significant number suffer with a double jeopardy—psoriasis combined with arthritis. Although the clinical features resemble other forms of arthritis, particularly rheumatoid, serological tests have a positive rheumatoid factor in rheumatoid arthritis but not necessarily so in psoriatic arthritis.

Experts cannot agree on the correlation between the incidence of psoriasis and arthritis. In his book, *Psoriasis*, Dr. Ronald Marks states: "Most surveys indicate that about 1 person in 20 with psoriasis has some form of arthritis, and that about 1 person in 20 with arthritis has some form of psoriasis."[1] According to a study by Gibble (1955), 2.5 to 5.5 percent of rheumatoid arthritis patients have psoriasis. Broad range estimates vary from less than 1 percent to 32 percent, presumably owing to the various definitions of arthritis.

Figures aside, the fact remains that the combination of the two problems, on the skin and in the joints, can create havoc with the patient and can, in the severe cases, lead to invalidism. Fortunately, these cases number relatively few among psoriatics, but they do occur and I have seen my fair share of them.

Psoriatic arthritis requires more work, patience, and discipline than any other form. For one thing, the patient probably began this disease process many years before starting treatment. It has been estimated that some patients have had skin lesions for 20 or 30 years before they started experiencing joint disease.

Psoriatic Arthritis has been recognized for about 100 years, and even in this form there are different classifications. For instance, there is *asymmetric oligoarthritis* which affects the majority of psoriatic arthritics (70%). "Oligo" means few or little joints, especially those in the hands near the knuckles. Then there is *symmetric polyarthritis* which closely resembles rheumatoid arthritis, but a blood test does not show a positive rheumatoid factor. This constitutes about 15% of those afflicted. *Polyarthritis* is a third form (about 5%) in which many joints are affected, usually near the fingertips and also in the feet. This type is considered the classic type of psoriatic arthritis. A fourth type is *psoriatic spondylitis* (also about 5%). In psoriatic spondylitis, the vertebrae are involved to a greater or lesser degree and should be of prime interest to the chiropractor or osteopath. More on this later in this chapter entitled "Poker Spine." The fifth type is *arthritis mutilans*. Again, only 5% of psoriatic arthritics are affected by it, but it is the most destructive type. In this there is bone destruction and deformity.

About Arthritis

Arthritis can strike anyone; it is no respecter of age. Its proportions range from minor aches or pains to complete incapacitation. Unless related directly to trauma or infection, its cause is largely unknown. But the one certainty common to most forms is inflamed joints.

The word arthritis is derived from the Greek prefix "arthron," meaning "pertaining to a joint;" and the suffix "itis," also from the Greek, meaning "inflammation." There are about a hundred forms of the disease, but by far the most common forms are rheumatoid arthritis (RA) and osteoarthritis (DJD—degenerative joint disease).

Approximately 36 million Americans are afflicted with arthritis with a million new cases occurring each year. Over 7 million arthritics have some disability and about 3 million are seriously impaired. Another report states there are 8 million people crippled with RA. Estimates show that three times more women than men contract this most serious form, even in childhood. Although the explanation for this "discrimination" is unknown, researchers are now questioning hormonal factors. In cases of psoriatic arthritis, however, the disease is found equally in men and women.

Virus Link?

A March 24, 1984, New York "Daily News" article by Judith Randal, "Link a virus to arthritis," related that scientists have succeeded in isolating a virus that may cause rheumatoid arthritis. Identified as the RA-1 virus, Dr. Robert Simpson, of the Waksman Institute of Microbiology at Rutgers University, feels this discovery may eventually lead to more effective treatment of the disease and possibly to a preventive vaccine. He also said his findings may make it possible to discover the cause of other diseases related to rheumatoid arthritis.

Since the features of psoriatic arthritis closely resemble those of rheumatoid arthritis, such as morning stiffness, pain on motion, tenderness, and swelling of small joints of the hands and feet, it behooves us to at least review some interesting Cayce concepts.

Same Problem—Different View

At first glance, it would appear that the present concept of viral invasion is worlds apart from the Cayce theory. A closer look, however, reveals they are not so far apart—they just differ in their basic premise.

It must be remembered that although viruses, bacteria, airborne and interior destructive elements surround us, most of them are rendered harmless in the healthy body. It is when the "healthy" body breaks down in some fashion that these destructive elements take over. Cayce claims that in arthritis, particularly rheumatoid, a high acidic nature of the body permits the virus or some other organism to thrive. It very well could be that the researchers at Rutgers University have isolated a virus relative to rheumatoid arthritis. The question remains, however, would this virus thrive in a different environment, i.e. one that is alkaline rather than acidic? Should efforts be centered on destroying the virus, or should they be concentrated on changing the internal environment of the host, that is, the body chemistry of the patient?

According to Cayce, maintaining alkalinity in the body, primarily through diet, will render a person virtually immune to such congestions. He particularly singled out lettuce, carrots, and celery as the most effective foods that help render the body alkaline.

If this be true, it follows that changing one's chemical, internal environment to alkaline is to ward off, prevent, or alleviate many arthritic conditions. Since this can be done primarily through diet and other safe methods, the research would not be so expensive or impractical. Some of my patients have done it on their own with excellent results. True, Cayce did not identify a specific virus as did Dr. Simpson and his associates at Rutgers. Nevertheless, Cayce's theory is not easily shrugged off when one considers the findings of Dr. Charles P. Lucas of the Wayne State University School of Medicine.

According to Dr. Lucas, who is also Chief of Endocrinology and Metabolism at Harper-Grace Hospitals, debilitating pain and severe joint swelling stemming from rheumatoid arthritis can be virtually eliminated when sufferers switch to a strict low-fat diet. A February 10, 1982, Associated Press article, "Low fat diet said to ease arthritis," quoted Dr. Lucas at a Detroit press conference. "I can't say that the low-fat diet is a cure, because as soon as patients go off that diet, their arthritis returns. But they can stay almost completely free of symptoms by eliminating fats from their diets."

Patients on the diet Dr. Lucas speaks of are allowed to eat whole wheat bread and cereals, vegetables, fruits, skim milk, rice, macaroni, and gelatin, among other foods, but are not allowed any meats other than salt-water fish. Except for one or two minor items, one would think his diet came right out of the Cayce archives.

If Cayce stressed anything about arthritis, or psoriasis, it was to *eliminate fats and eat many fresh fruits and vegetables.*

The psoriatic arthritic must also be very mindful of avoiding salt and salted products, in particular. Just a pat of light salted butter can flare up swollen ankles or wrists to a marked degree. When one particular patient substituted a little sweet butter for the salted butter, a decided difference was experienced immediately. She then took the time to read labels and avoided salted products as much as possible. In her particular case, the swelling of the ankles and wrists diminished in a matter of days; walking was much easier, and generalized aches and pains subsided to an appreciable degree.

This same patient substituted skim milk for whole milk, because the whole milk variety contains salt as well as fat. Ice cream also has salt and fat in it, so she used yogurt. She selected the low fat, low salt or no salt cheeses. Her body was becoming her servant rather than the other way around. Why? Because she took the *time* to study her own reactions, read labels, and even be creative in solving her own problems.

Further research on the effects certain foods have on arthritis is revealed in the works of Dr. Norman F. Childers of the University of Florida and founder of the Nightshades Research Foundation. As stated earlier, he has undeniably traced the adverse effects the nightshade family of plants have on the arthritic. His prescription is *The No-Nightshade Diet*. His research is gaining in popularity with patients as well as their physicians.

If one were to combine the findings of Dr. Lucas and Dr. Childers and add a touch of Cayce, a formula evolves to ward off arthritis as well as psoriasis. Eliminate fats, the nightshades, sweets, and alcohol. Drink plenty of fresh water. Eat large quantities of fresh fruits and select vegetables. Fish, fowl or lamb, are permitted, but nothing fried. Cayce, obviously, is even more lenient than the researchers in allowing fowl and lamb. Nevertheless, in the vast majority of cases, given adequate time, it works.

A Picture Evolves

The discourses of Edgar Cayce never included a file per se on the disease entity *psoriatic arthritis*. There is available, however, quite an extensive treatise on the individual conditions, psoriasis and arthritis. As a matter of fact, these two conditions are among the top ten circulating files most frequently requested by the over 100,000 members of the Cayce Foundation.

Careful study of both files reveals a close similarity in managing both these conditions. Common sense dictates that a combination of the therapeutic regimens for psoriasis and rheumatoid arthritis is the best and most reasonable course to follow. My advice to my patients with psoriatic arthritis is:

1. Follow the psoriasis regimen to the letter.

2. Add the following measures derived from the discourses on rheumatoid arthritis.

    a) A full body peanut oil massage twice a week if possible. Leave the oil on for at least 1/2 hour after the massage before washing it off. Shower down, but do not use soap. Some patients leave the oils on overnight.

    b) A peanut oil tub bath. To a tub of comfortably hot water, add one cup of cold pressed peanut oil. Submerge up to the neck and remain at least 1/2 hour. As the water cools, add additional hot water.

CAUTION: Peanut oil baths leave the tub very slippery. The patients must be sure to have someone help them in and out of the tub. After the bath, they pat themselves dry, leaving the light coating of peanut oil on over-night. Obviously, it's best to do this just before bedtime.

c) Add Jerusalem artichokes (Sunchokes) to the diet, once a week.

d) Avoid bananas and strawberries.

e) Eat all kinds of raw vegetables (except cabbage) in *Knox Gelatin*. These may include watercress, chard, mustard greens, kale, carrots, celery, lettuce (leaf or romaine). These vegetables must be prepared *within* the gelatin—as a gelatin salad. As mentioned in my chapter, "Diet and Nutrition," gelatin has been called a catalyst in the body, helping it to better absorb the vitamins and other properties of fruits and vegetables.

f) Cleansing of the colon by high colonic irrigations or high enemas play a significant role in alleviating arthritis. Colonics or high enemas should be used approximately every 10 days from the beginning of therapy for at least two months. Thereafter, perhaps once a month until all symptoms subside—then about four times a year, at the change of seasons.

g) No alcoholic drinks.

Since rheumatoid arthritis is so closely tied to psoriatic arthritis, the same precautionary measures apply. Do not disturb the body too greatly and more time is to be expected as part of the regimen. The course to follow in psoriatic arthritic cases is the slow, gentle approach.

The above measures are those that I found most practical. A most informative treatise on both arthritis and psoriasis is found in the *Physician's Reference Notebook*, compiled and edited by William A. McGarey, M.D., Director of the Medical Research Division and published by the A.R.E. Press. This volume, once only available to licensed physicians, is now available to the public through the A.R.E. Bookstore, Virginia Beach, VA 23451.

Avoiding "Winter Itch" (Asteatotic Dermatitis)

The psoriatic arthritic patients I have encountered seem to be more affected by the itch with tightening and cracking of the skin in winter months than does the patient who has only psoriasis to contend with. This is due to the lack of moisture in the skin and is caused by the dry environment in the household that occurs when turning on the heat.

Two of the best remedies for this problem are mentioned in my chapter, "External Applications," under the heading, "Physiotherapy at home." They are the whirlpool and the humidifier.

A home whirlpool treatment, using comfortably hot water for approximately twenty minutes, followed by a gentle peanut oil massage, will not only feel comforting but will also help retain moisture in the skin.

In winter, Epsom salts baths are generally avoided as it tends to dry out the skin too much. I do advise, however, to add 1/2 to 1 cup of peanut oil to the water while the whirlpool is operating. After the prescribed amount of time, the patient carefully emerges from the tub, pats skin dry and relaxes.

They remember to observe the necessary precautions. They do not use a whirlpool if they suffer from a heart condition of any kind. They make certain that there is someone on hand in the event of a fainting spell and also to lend assistance in getting in and out of the tub.

A humidifier is extremely helpful in keeping the air in the room moist, especially while sleeping. Breathing in moist air avoids drawing moisture from the skin and allows the surface cells to remain pliable. Thorough cleansing of these units daily is essential to prevent spores from forming that may become airborne, potentially causing respiratory ailments. Several brands now have the means of preventing this from happening. Instructions are provided by the manufacturer.

Again, both a portable home whirlpool and humidifier are readily available in department stores at a nominal cost. I consider them a wise investment for the psoriatic arthritic.

Stress and Its Effects

Since the cause of arthritis is unknown and the cause of psoriasis is unknown (from the orthodox point of view), it naturally follows that the cause of psoriatic arthritis is likewise unknown. I am often prone to follow a simple rule in trying to get at the bottom of a patient's condition. That rule is—ask the patient! In my opinion, every physician should ask his patient, "What do you think is the cause of your condition?" Some of the answers are amazing. And even more astonishing is to see how accurate the patient can be when a diagnosis is finally reached.

It seems to me, in the case of psoriatic arthritis, based on a number of cases I have seen through the years, that *stressful living conditions* heads the list of possible basic causes.

I have had a good number of severely afflicted straight psoriasis or straight arthritic cases who live under ideal conditions (at least from outward appearances). On the other hand, I have rarely, if ever, found a psoriatic arthritic case who lived without stressful conditions as part of their life-style. Of course, the question, "What came first—the chicken or the egg?" may be asked. In other words, did the stressful living conditions cause the illness, or did the illness bring about stressful living conditions?

Regardless of what came first, there was a slow, but steady buildup of toxins in the body before the victim found that he or she could not get out of bed one morning.

I cannot help but feel that negative attitudes and emotions play a significant role in these cases, creating stress, tension, up-tightness, and all that goes with it—even though there may be some justification in harboring such attitudes.

Anger, for instance, is only one of the negative states of mind that lends itself to creating a stressful atmosphere. Others are: fear, jealousy, loneliness, insecurity (financial or otherwise), job pressure (either actual or imaginary), inharmonious family, and other similar situations, all of which can come up with the same end result—a sick body formed by a sick soul.

Miss D.K.'s Story

Miss D.K. was a lovely young school teacher suffering with psoriatic arthritis when she first visited my office on July 26, 1985. She had been in this state of ill health since adolescence and knew full well that stress was largely responsible for her condition. In the following discourse, she describes her plight and eventual triumph.

"Getting psoriatic arthritis was the best thing that ever happened to me because of all I've learned.

"I was the youngest child born into a home replete with alcoholism, anger, and violence. There were so many rules and regulations, I had to keep so much inside. I spent most of my time alone up in my third floor bedroom extremely depressed. I felt I had been born into the wrong family. I had contemplated suicide on and off since I'd been 8 years old. Frequently throughout my childhood, I would wake up during the night with excruciating pain in my legs and arms. I suspect my parents didn't believe me as they never took me to the doctor, but instructed me to drink milk, thinking I was not getting enough calcium or whatever.

"One Sunday, when I was in the eight grade (the prime of my adolescence), my legs swelled up like watermelons. Trips to several doctors left me undiagnosed. 'She'll grow out of it,' they said.

"Boy, was I miserable. I was fat and lonely with swollen legs, trying to 'fit in' by wearing the super short dresses that were in vogue during the late sixties; not to mention the fact that my face was breaking out. Even though I relied on my Catholicism (church was my place of solace) I knew my life was not happening at random. I always felt I had somehow done something to earn all this, and that there was good to be gained in some way.

"In high school, I attracted some nice friends and even a boyfriend by senior year. Things were looking up.

"At age 19, I met the person who introduced me to the philosophy of Edgar Cayce. Something inside me clicked. It was all so beautiful, and at least I had reasonable answers to my life's situations. And yes, I was responsible. But my life would get worse before it got better.

"My 'turbulent twenties' consisted of several up and down relationships with men, a drinking problem, a severe case of psoriasis, and then the accompanying arthritis. There was definitely something wrong.

"I really hit bottom at age twenty-eight. A strong relationship with a man ended abruptly, my arthritis was so bad I couldn't move (medication wasn't helping), and consequently I was forced to leave my waitressing job. (I was also teaching part-time, but most of my income came from the restaurant job.) Financially, I was down to minus dollars and I was supporting myself. I spent count-less hours sitting alone in my apartment reading Edgar Cayce's *'Think On These Things'* and other spiritual as well as medical material.

"I did get a new full-time teaching position, which enabled me to afford counseling. I slowly started to improve—my joints were working again, but the psoriasis persisted.

"While attending a conference at A.R.E., I saw photos of Dr. Pagano's work, and once again, something clicked. I became his patient, and by following his recommendations, my psoriasis has almost disappeared. Not only that, but I feel stronger and happier every day.

"Now at age thirty-one, my life is going uphill. I have wonderful friends, a very pleasant job with financial stability, and a renewed interest in life."   D.K.

When people meet Miss D.K. today, they think she was born with a smile on her face, an enthusiasm for life, and a positive outlook for the future. Little do they know of the internal turmoil and strain she experi-enced. She took the action step by studying, meditating, contemplating, and visualizing in order to bring about the changes desired. Today she is an inspiration to all her students, friends, and especially to my new psori-asis patients with whom she has agreed to meet and offer encouragement.

I cite this case because of the similarity I have found with other psori-atic arthritics. D.K. also has proven to herself that a change of mind also helps change the chemistry of the body—but as in all things worth-while—it takes a commitment. There is no substitute for time, patience, and persistence.

Atomodine

No account of the Edgar Cayce approach to arthritis, particularly the rheumatoid type, would be complete without mentioning a substance called Atomodine. It is called for in several systemic conditions especially in the long standing, degenerative type diseases like psoriatic arthritis.

As a chiropractic physician, I cannot personally prescribe the use of Atomodine, for to do so borders on practicing medicine. I only mention the substance's existence for those readers and researchers who might not have heard of it before. In such cases, I therefore advise my patients to first consult with a medical doctor or osteopath regarding the use of Atomodine. *Under no circumstances should Atomodine be used without medical approval.* One drop of it supplies about six times the minimum daily requirement of iodine, and too much iodine can lead to over stimulation of the thyroid gland, resulting in nervousness, insomnia, and rapid heartbeat. A person allergic to even the smallest amount of iodine can have a severe reaction. Nevertheless, approximately 610 Cayce readings enthusiastically mention Atomodine in cases involving glandular deficiency or malfunction associated with a shortage of iodine in the system.

One of the many recommendations for its use was to take it internally for cases of arthritis. Its purpose is to "purify" the glands, and it often called for taking only one drop of Atomodine in half a glass of water a few days out of the week, then skipping it for about a week, then beginning again. Different patients were offered different suggestions on how much to take. That is why the substance cannot be used indiscriminately. I found it quite interesting to discover some readings stating that, for most effectiveness, spinal adjustments are to be given in conjunction with the taking of Atomodine.

Atomodine, or "atomic iodine," is valuable because it is iodine in a form apparently less toxic to the body than the molecular iodine generally available in Kelp tablets, or Lugol's Solution.

Atomodine was rarely prescribed as a treatment by itself, but was to be used as a part of various programs also involving other important measures.*

Glyco-Thymoline

Keeping in mind that the underlying common denominator for the psoriatic arthritic is to reduce acidity and promote alkalinity of the body, the use of the substance Glyco-Thymoline taken internally (just a few-drops in a glass of water) holds an honored place when it comes to internal purification, as does Atomodine.

---

*Members of the A.R.E. can obtain more precise details on Atomodine by consulting the appropriate Circulating File. The A.R.E. publication, "An Edgar Cayce Home Medicine Guide," available to the general public, carries a very informative article on Atomodine. A.R.E. Bookstore, Box 595, Virginia Beach, VA 23451.

Glyco-Thymoline, a mouth wash, is useful to the psoriatic, not only from an internal point of view in that it cleanses and purifies the intestinal tract, but it is also an anti-pruritic (reduces itching) when used externally. Applied full strength to the irritated areas, it often works when all else fails. Since itching is a major problem for patients, it is helpful for the patient to keep a bottle of the alkaline formula handy. For the genital areas, I recommend a warm sitz bath with a mixture of 1/3 to 1/2 or as much as a full bottle (16 oz.) of Glyco-Thymoline added to 3-4 gallons of comfortably hot water—about 102 degrees Fahrenheit.

Therefore, there are only three substances within the Edgar Cayce Regimen for psoriasis and/or arthritis that should be first approved by a medical doctor or osteopath. They are: Atomodine, Glyco-Thymoline and the Tri-Salts Compound (Sulphur, Cream of Tartar and Rochelle Salts) which we covered in my chapter "Internal Cleansing." Again, they are non-prescription items and may be obtained from the Cayce product suppliers (Appendix C), but since they are to be taken internally, they should be approved by practitioners licensed in dispensing drugs.

Swollen Joints

When the joints of the body become severely swollen and inflamed, the psoriatic arthritic becomes practically incapacitated. The pain can be excruciating, movement extremely limited, and weight-bearing next to impossible. When the ankles in particular are affected, it is most devastating, obviously, because of the restrictions this places on the patient in getting from one place to another.

Any joint or number of joints can be affected; ankles, small bones of the feet, knees, hip joints, shoulders, wrists, and small bones of the hand. In the chapter, "Psoriasis of the Hands and Feet," a very effective treatment is outlined. In the case of psoriatic arthritis of these areas, the therapy is similar.

All things being equal, that is, diet, colonics or enemas, water intake, etc., the use of hot soaks of Epsom Salts followed by peanut oil massage into the joints, has been found to be extremely helpful.

Patients are advised to make a hot Epsom salt solution by adding one half to one pound of the salts to a basin or bowl which should be 3/4 full of hot water. If the hands are being treated, they soak the hands and wrists in the water for five minutes, working the wrists in various directions.

They massage the hands together under water, working the fingers and rotating the joints, soak again for another five or ten minutes, then pat dry. At this point, they rub 100 percent pure cold-pressed peanut oil throughout the hands, wrists, and up the arm. They then place hands in disposable, plastic or plain cotton gloves which can be purchased at any discount beauty supply shop or drugstore. The gloves are left on for at least an hour, often over-night. This same basic procedure is used for the ankles and feet, but a large "baggie" is used in place of gloves covered by a white sock. Many patients have reported using a baggie and a white sock for their hands as well in place of gloves, and, again, many use only a white sock without the baggies. Whatever is more comfortable should be used. By using knee-high gym socks they can cover the entire hand, wrist, and lower arm—up to the elbow which often has visible lesions.

If one has a small whirlpool designed for the hands and feet, such as the Oster, I recommend they use this every other day. Some peanut oil can be placed in the water of the massage unit. After use, there may be a problem lifting up the unit to empty out the water. If there is no one handy to do it, it can be done simply by using a quart size container and emptying the water bucket by bucket. Although awkward, it is better than not using the unit at all.

Hot Epsom Salts packs are also very helpful for swollen joints. This is accomplished by soaking a small terrycloth towel in hot water and saturating it heavily with Epsom Salts. After squeezing excess water out of the towel, it is wrapped around the joint being treated, covered with plastic wrap, then an electric (waterproof) heating pad is placed around the entire setup. In cases involving the wrist, knees, elbows, and ankles, the Gillette "wraparound" electric heat unit, or something similar, is most effective.

I advise my patients to leave it on low or medium heat for about twenty minutes, or what seems comfortable to them. When they unravel the heating unit, they are to massage peanut oil into the joint.

At times, I have recommended rubbing warm peanut oil on the joint first, then placing the Epsom salt pack over it with the heating pad.

Admittedly, this is a bit of a bother, but once the routine is established, it becomes second nature—especially when the patient begins to feel better.

An example of the effectiveness of these procedures was published in Dr. McGarey's quarterly newsletter "Pathways to Health," where he describes his success with one of his patients as follows:

"Case History—Rheumatoid Arthritis ....

"Two years ago, Fred showed up at the Clinic with a three-month history of swelling and redness in his right foot and ankle, and recent development of back pain. He had been tested for rheumatoid arthritis and the latest test returned positive. Fred was 65. Aside from these things, he had been in excellent health.

"His regimen of therapy followed very closely the suggestions given in the readings and in the Circulating File on this condition; Atomodine in series and in cycles, Epsom salts baths each week, full-body massages while at the Clinic to be followed by local massages with peanut oil on his foot and ankle each night before retiring, visualization techniques, and an arthritis diet.

"His response was rapid. In two months, the swelling was gone, there was no discomfort and no stiffness, and, to all intents and purposes, he was well."[2]

It must not be assumed, however, that the coexistence of psoriatic lesions and joint pain automatically labels the diagnosis psoriatic arthritis. It may be a simultaneous condition of gout, rheumatoid arthritis, or even systemic lupus erythematosus. In these less typical cases, serological tests for the rheumatoid factor and a LE cell preparation should be made medically which may assist in establishing a diagnosis.

From an x-ray point of view, the most striking histopathologic alteration in psoriatic arthritis are the destructive bone changes near the joint surface and in the adjacent shaft. An x-ray of the small joints of the hands and feet is often helpful in evaluating the extent of the disease. The radiologist would look for signs of erosion of osseous (bone) tissue, particularly in the distal phalangeal joints (fingertips), as well as destruction of bone in the metatarsal and interphalangeal joints of the feet.

These are all clinical findings and are really the concern of the diagnostician. The point made here for the patient is to recognize the fact that pain throughout the joints, combined with psoriasis, does not necessarily spell out psoriatic arthritis. More than likely it is, but it may also mean that there is an underlying condition present which is incidental to their psoriasis. Nevertheless, the treatment is basically the same, whether or not they are combined or separate conditions.

Poker Spine

One of the most disabling symptoms occurs when psoriatic arthritis affects the spine—which, in my practice, has been the case with a good number of patients. Of course, there are varying degrees of spinal involvement. The types I have encountered most frequently are those in which there is practically no flexibility of the spine. Thus the term "poker spine." It is like trying to manipulate a steel rod. This is a characteristic feature of conditions known as Rheumatoid Arthritis of the spine, Spondyloarthritis, Ankylosing Spondylitis, and Psoriatic Spondylitis.

In long standing cases, the spine on x-ray examination may look like a calcified steel rod—or—it may be unremarkable. Either way, the normal range of motion, flexibility, and pliability of the spine is absent. The longitudinal spinal ligaments and soft tissue elements surrounding the vertebrae are so dried up and rigid that movement, even by manipulation, is virtually impossible.

Age has little to do with it. I have patients in their twenties just as rigid as others with the same problem who are in their sixties.

In this, the chiropractor or the osteopath must exercise extreme caution by not being too forceful in their downward pressure in an attempt to achieve movement of the spinal motor units. Gentle, steady downward pressure all along the spine, without attempting to adjust anything, is the procedure I follow. We are aiming for improved flexibility, not spinal correction. It is all that can be expected anyway and the patients will love their practitioner for being gentle in their approach. In time, with the steady use of peanut oil massages, particularly along the spine, the doctor may feel minor adjustments taking place. With continued conservative manipulation, more flexibility will be established and, in time, a greater range of motion, without pain, will be experienced by the patient.

In cases of this severity, treatment must be expected to continue for a year or more, which is nothing when one considers the alternative. At least something is being done about it that will help put the condition in check and slowly reverse the disease process. Doing nothing invariably means a continued lifetime of pain with increasing immobility leading to possible invalidism.

Some Added Measures

The bottom line in psoriatic arthritis is time, patience, and effort. There is no substitute. It must be remembered that the patient's chemistry is out of balance—even if the myriad of serological tests show negative results. Here is a case where the patient's reaction serves as the best barometer in determining the degree of progress.

Since these cases fall within the most severe type of psoriasis known, every form of hydrotherapy (water therapy) should be utilized: steam, whirlpool, colonics, fume baths, swimming, (See Chapter—"External Applications") and yes, one can consider drinking 6 to 8 tumblers of pure water as part of "internal" hydrotherapy.

Controlled modalities such as electrical stimulation, as well as roller type massage units along the entire spine can be extremely helpful.

Gentle stretch exercises are encouraged but must be geared to the patient in each case. Sustained stretch positions, such as yoga postures, are very helpful and therapeutic. They also provide a criteria to judge improvement by increased range of motion.

Finally, as a mental exercise, key words should be visualized and even uttered audibly to oneself. Words that signify where they want to go, such as: Flexibility, Rubber, Elastic, Stretchability, Raggedy Ann, "Loose as a goose," etc.

These power pack words have more significance than one may think. They represent an attitude—one that is the very opposite of what psoriatic arthritis represents. I advise my patients to "Try it—you might like it."

Loosen Up!

And last, but by no means least, I advise my patients with this form of the disease to start *taking things lightly*. I tell them to start loosening up mentally as well as physically, learn to bend with the wind, and don't be so harsh on themselves or others. The reasoning behind such attitudes is simple when one realizes the eternal truth that *a rigid mentality has as its constant companion—a rigid body!*

REFERENCES

(Chapter 15—The Arthritic Connection)

1. Dr. Ronald Marks, *Psoriasis*, (New York, NY, Arco Publishing, Inc., © 1981, p. 32.)
2. *Pathways to Health*—June/July 1979, Medical Research Bulletin. Volume 1, Number 2. The A.R.E. Clinic—4018 North 40th Street, Phoenix, Arizona 85018.

Chapter 16

A Case of Eczema

The disease that comes closest in simulating psoriasis is eczema. Both produce scales, have reddened, inflamed areas, "ooze" at times, and can produce an uncontrollable itch that is a living hell for the patient.

From the orthodox medical viewpoint, they are considered two separate diseases. From a medical therapy point of view, this is probably best because the treatments differ. From the Edgar Cayce readings, however, we learn the exact opposite. There most certainly is a correlation between the two diseases, not only in cause, but also in treatment.

During my years of working with psoriasis, a few cases of eczema came into the office. Admittedly, this hardly constitutes a basis for a valid research report, but when three out of four clear up completely by basically following the same regimen I give for psoriasis, something here demands our attention.

The First Case:

In December 1979, Mr. R.P. came to me complaining of a severe case of eczema. Having suffered with it for years, he desperately sought a remedy. He had heard of my work with psoriasis through the A.R.E. and wondered if I could offer any help. I made it quite clear at our first meeting that I had never encountered a case of eczema and had no experience with it. However, his desperate plea touched me and I agreed to send for the Cayce file on eczema with the understanding that I would not take the case if the therapy did not fall within my scope of practice. With this understanding, we proceeded.

Amazingly, a careful perusal of the eczema discourses revealed such a startling parallel to psoriasis that I was almost convinced they had sent the wrong file! Not so; it *was* the eczema file. For two weeks I studied and extracted every possible measure that could benefit Mr. P.

The cause of eczema was listed as the same thinning of the intestinal walls, a super-toxic body accompanied by poor elimination. The adherence to a high alkaline diet was essential with proper elimination as the key factor in treatment. Only one external measure, the application of Ray's Ointment or Liquid or Lenoir's Eczema Remedy, was suggested often for eczema and only occasionally for psoriasis. Since they are not prescription items, the patient obtained them on his own. The same Slippery Elm Powder, Saffron and Mullein Tea were the primary herbs suggested for intestinal cleansing. The adjustments of the spine were slightly different: the emphasis was placed on the 3rd and 4th dorsal area, throughout the lumbars, but did also have special reference to the 6th dorsal. The similarity in cause and treatment of eczema and psoriasis was all too apparent in the Cayce material.

After placing Mr. P. on the same basic regimen as for psoriasis, the patient agreed to follow each measure as faithfully as possible. He came to my office for a few visits, but then was unable to return for three months. When he did return, the results were more than encouraging. For the first time in years he was enthusiastic, vital, vibrant, and his skin had improved considerably.

Within another month, all discomfort had subsided. Within six months he was satisfied with the condition of his skin and in all other areas of his life as well. His job endeavors improved slowly but steadily, his skin remained clear, his attitude was extremely positive, and the sense of desperation and anxiety had given way to one of calmness. He was a relaxed man, in charge of his life again.

On October 29, 1980, I gave a talk on psoriasis in the Dag Hammarskold Library Auditorium at the United Nations in New York. As I prepared to go on stage, Mr. P. came up to inform me that he was in the audience, and if I cared to mention his particular case, he would confirm it. An opportunity toward the end of the talk opened up and his case was presented. After I introduced him, he surprised everybody, including me, by exposing his arms and legs now totally clear of eczema, confirming his success by following the regimen.

I had no way of knowing whether or not this treatment would work in all cases of eczema; but, in his case, thanks to his self-discipline, it worked indeed.

In the two years following the case of Mr. P., I only had two other cases of eczema. One was an adorable little black girl whose mother followed all instructions conscientiously to another successful outcome. Another was an adult black women suffering from a very severe case of eczema since infancy. I do not consider her response successful, although she improved somewhat after three to four months. She discontinued further treatment in favor of other methods. Perhaps more time was needed to cleanse her body internally. One thing however, stands out in her case history—she had had a lifetime of poor elimination.

A Case Via Telephone

It wasn't until January 1983 that I encountered the next case of eczema. One weekend Alice G., a dear friend of mine from upstate New York, related to me the sad plight of her life-long friend, Mrs. M.K., who was ninety-two years old. Mrs. M.K. had been a very active person until 1981 when she developed a very harsh case of eczema. The itch throughout her arms was unbearable. Although she had been under the care of two dermatologists during this time, nothing brought her relief and the condition worsened.

Alice asked me if there was anything I could do for her. I answered it was possible, providing she followed all instructions. Alice insisted that I call her and discuss the matter as she was in a desperate state. The voice on the phone was that of a marvelous human being with a deep-rooted, loving philosophy of life that had sustained her positively through the years. Her gratitude for my time was apparent from the beginning of the conversation. She explained that she had been diagnosed by both her dermatologists as having eczema. Even at the age of ninety-two, she would not accept this as her fate or destiny. She knew there was an answer somewhere.

Since the case of Mr. R.P. proved so successful, I was able to convey to her the details of his success as well as my experience with psoriasis. A leading researcher, considered to be an authority on psoriasis, has said: "It is not much good treating someone for psoriasis if what they have is really eczema." This probably holds true from the viewpoint of orthodox treatment, but from the Cayce outlook, I must answer this fine physician with the fact that I have found the opposite to be true.

As I dictated the regimen to Mrs. M.K. over the phone, she took detailed notes, and not once, but three or four times, repeated how grateful she was and that she would follow it to the letter. When I explained the importance of proper elimination, in that there should be no constipation at all, she sighed with relief. She explained, "I told the doctors that I was often constipated, but they would virtually ignore me and made it sound unimportant and unrelated to my problem." I suggested that she take the necessary steps to relieve her constipation problem, post haste.

In addition, and equally important, I took her off whole milk and placed her on goat's milk. The powdered form is found, or can be ordered, in most health food stores. This determined, enthusiastic woman followed every suggestion to the best of her ability. She sent out for the proper vegetables, juices, herb teas, etc. Within the first month, the condition worsened as often happens even in psoriasis cases. Then slowly, a change began to occur. A gradual, steady improvement manifested as the change of diet helped regulate the bowel movements, and elimination was no longer a problem.

The few times her visiting nurse administered a home enema made a decided difference. I advised a regulated diet, especially one which avoids foods with a high-fat content and which excluded nightshades or sweets. Goat's milk became a regular part of her diet. The regimen paid off handsomely, but her desire to rid her own body of this irritating disease was the overriding factor.

The next time I heard from Mrs. K. was in the spring of 1983 while I was visiting Alice, five months after our initial telephone conversation. Mrs. K. insisted that I visit her. This I did, and I am happy to relate that a joyful, dignified, elegant lady greeted me at the door. There wasn't a mark or lesion on her. She now enjoyed freedom from that unbearable itch, pain and stiffness.

She had invited me to visit her not only to see first hand the results obtained but also to thank me personally for putting her on the right track. In appreciation, she gave me one of her prized possessions, a 1936 edition of *Gone With the Wind*, signed by the author, Margaret Mitchell, who had been a personal friend of the family. She endorsed it over to me on the first page with "To Dr. John Pagano, with deep gratitude for curing me of eczema—June 4, 1983."

Her story is an inspiration to me and all who know her. A woman of ninety-two, instead of "throwing in the towel," made up her mind to do whatever was required. After receiving instructions, by only a phone call or two, she was determined to follow through, and she succeeded. For those younger patients with eczema who feel the procedure is too much trouble, I have only pity. The road ahead can be long, tedious, expensive, and a great deal of pain and effort by not considering this alternative.

I visited Mrs. K. again in August 1983 on her invitation to choose all the books I wanted from her library. Before departing her gracious company, I asked the one proverbial question, "Mrs. K., what do you believe was the key to getting well?" She thought a moment and, with a twinkle in her eye, looked up at me and said, "Well, doctor, eloquently speaking, when I stopped being constipated!"

In 1987, I gave a lecture in northern New Jersey to an audience in which a medical doctor was present. She was quite moved by the evidence I presented as well as meeting some patients themselves. It wasn't long before she referred a severe case of eczema to me. The patient, Mr. R.U., in his late twenties suffered with eczema from across his shoulders up into his entire head. He looked as though he had dipped his head and shoulders into a bucket of light red paint. No other parts of his body were affected. All measures used for psoriasis were employed—but he noticed the biggest change when he eliminated tomatoes and vinegar from his diet. He was totally free of the problem in less than four months. The itch, which was absolutely intolerable, was the first symptom to go. Today (1990) he remains free of the problem.

Another case, that of Mrs. G.M., followed the diet and all other measures and was quite pleased at the progress being made except for the fact that the eczema flared up every night while in bed for no apparent reason. One night she visited a friend and stayed over night. She did not experience any adverse reaction when sleeping in the guest's bedroom. When she returned home and slept in her own bed there was again a flare-up. Upon careful questioning, we determined what the culprit was. At her friend's home she slept in a bed with linen sheets. Her own bed always had silk sheets, which did not allow her skin to "breathe" as easily as did the cotton fabric. When she changed over to linen or cotton sheets and pillow cases, results were immediately apparent.

The case of Mrs. G.M. led to our advising cotton fabric on not only bed sheets, but pajamas and undergarments, especially panty hose. Even bathing suits are best when made of cotton (or a large percentage of it) rather than nylon, silk or rubberized. In other words, the eczema or psoriatic will do well to avoid any synthetic fabric clinging to the skin. The more the skin can breathe, the better the results.

The reader should have a clear appreciation of the similarities in cause and regimen of treatment for psoriasis and eczema. There are, however, a few specific differences in treating eczema as compared to psoriasis. The regimen is basically the same except for the external application of Ray's Ointment for Eczema vs. Cuticura or Hydrophilic Ointment for Psoriasis. Internally, as an intestinal cleanser, any good natural laxative will do; such as, stewed fruits, syrup of figs, Senokot, Psyllium Husks, etc. The only stipulation here is to try to alternate using a laxative with a fruit base at one time with one having a vegetable base at another time. It is best not to use the same type of laxative all the time.

Other differences are minor; but, for the reader's interest, I have listed below a comparative view of both conditions followed by some appropriate dietary measures.

CORRELATION BETWEEN PSORIASIS & ECZEMA

PSORIASIS	*ECZEMA*
(Gk., p<u>sora</u>, the itch)	(Gk. <u>ek</u> + zeo, boil)
1. Basically a toxemia	1. Basically a toxemia

2. Cause: Poor elimination
   Thinning of intestinal walls
	2. Cause: Poor elimination
	   Thinning of intestinal walls

3. Blood: Excess acidity	3. Blood: Excess acidity
4. Cathartics (Laxatives):	4. Cathartics (Laxatives):
a. Innerclean	a. Innerclean
b. Senokot	b. Senokot
c. Olive Oil	c. Olive Oil
d. Psyllium Husks	d. Psyllium Husks
e. Milk of Magnesia	e. Milk of Magnesia
f. Fletcher's Castoria	f. Fletcher's Castoria

5. External applications:
   a. Cuticura Ointment
   b. Castor Oil
   c. Hydrophilic Ointment
   d. Olive Oil/Peanut Oil

6. Spinal Adjustments:
   (in order of importance)
   a. 6th, 7th & 9th Dorsal
   b. 3rd Cervical
   c. Throughout the Lumbars, especially the 4th

7. Sources of irritation:
   a. Duodenum
   b. Jejunum
   c. Upper intestinal tract

8. Recommended:
   High colonic irrigations followed by Glyco-Thymoline (diluted) as a final rinse
   Home enemas

9. Diet should be highly alkaline

10. Fish, Fowl & Lamb (never fried) is permitted

11. No alcohol (Red wine as a food is ok)

12. Skim or low fat milk and/or buttermilk is permitted

13. Drink six to eight glasses of pure water daily

14. Sunshine usually helps but not always

5. External applications:
   a. Ray's Ointment
   b. Lenoir's Eczema Remedy
   c. Olive Oil/Peanut Oil

6. Spinal Adjustments:
   (in order of importance)
   a. 3rd, 4th, 6th & 9th Dorsal
   b. 3rd Cervical
   c. Throughout the Lumbars, especially the 4th

7. Sources of irritation:
   a. Stomach
   b. Duodenum/Jejunum
   c. Upper intestinal tract

8. Recommended:
   High colonic irrigations followed by Glyco-Thymoline (diluted) as a final rinse
   Home enemas

9. Diet should be highly alkaline

10. Fowl & Lamb, Occasionally Fish (never fried), well masticated, is permitted

11. No alcohol (Red wine as a food is ok)

12. Goat's Milk or Soy Milk is preferred.

13. Drink six to eight glasses of pure water daily

14. Sunshine is usually harmful

15. Undergarments and bed linens should be made of cotton or should have a high cotton content.

16. If on hands, wear protective gloves when washing dishes or working with solvents

15. Undergarments and bed linens should be made of cotton or should have a high cotton content.

16. If on hands, wear protective gloves when washing dishes or working with solvents

<u>NOTE</u>: Products such as, Innerclean, Ray's Ointment, Olive Oil/Peanut Oil mixture and Glyco-Thymoline can be obtained through the Cayce Suppliers listed in Appendix C.

Red wine is not permitted if any type of adverse reaction occurs, such as itching, or if the patient also has gout or is on medication.

FACTORS IN COMMON: PSORIASIS/ECZEMA

1. Eat plenty of green leafy vegetables, especially watercress, celery and lettuce.

2. Saffron Tea and Mullein Tea called for in both. Plenty of water. No carbonated drinks.

3. The perspiratory glands become more active in both cases when there is a lack of coordination in the eliminating system, therefore, synthetic undergarments, especially those that cling to the skin, are to be avoided. Preferred are undergarments, as well as bed linens, made of cotton or those that have a high percentage of cotton in their composition.

4. Maintain a cheerful disposition. Smile—even if it takes the hide off—for to worry or become cross and antagonistic creates poisons, just as much as, or even more so, than the wrong foods.

5. Slippery Elm Bark Powder in water every other morning is a good general rule for both.

6. Independent research has proven that two to four tablespoons of lecithin (granular) each day is extremely helpful in both psoriasis and eczema.

7. No nightshades in either case, especially tomatoes, and hot spices, no vinegar, no shellfish. Animal fats should be cut down considerably. Fish, fowl and lamb are permitted—but never fried. The dietary measures for eczema in general are the same as those suggested for psoriasis. *It cannot be overemphasized that diet and internal cleansing are the key factors in alleviating eczema as well as psoriasis.*

I have no answer as to why one person gets eczema while another gets psoriasis if the cause is the same. That can only be determined by detailed scientific investigation, if at all. Perhaps they are different forms of the same disease, but someone in authority placed labels on them and, as a result, they are viewed as different diseases. Such a precept can put one off the track from the start.

One factor of considerable importance which characterizes the study of the Cayce material is that several different diseases are basically treated the same way with satisfactory results reported in many cases. This seems to be especially true in the classification of degenerative diseases such as psoriasis, arthritis, scleroderma, and other systemic problems. It is as though the body is telling us, "Set me right, feed me correctly, expect me to get well and I'll heal myself."

It has been my experience to treat a number of these *seemingly* different health problems. The basic principles of the psoriasis regimen were followed and a successful outcome was often the result. In the next chapter, a few such cases are presented along with some interesting stories on psoriasis.

Chapter 17

Some Interesting Cases

Every physician, regardless of his specialty, experiences cases which stand out in his memory. My years of caring for psoriatics have left me with many fond, and some not so fond, memories and bits of knowledge gleaned only from practical firsthand experience.

My Introduction to Psoriasis

I met Mr. H. while interning in Denver, Colorado. Until then, my knowledge of psoriasis was limited to textbook photographs and descriptions. There, for the first time, I saw psoriasis "in the flesh."

"Covered from head to toe" is the only way to describe Mr. H.'s condition. Throughout his life he had been unsuccessfully searching for help. His desperate plea aroused my interest to the point where I began gathering all available information I could on this disease. It marked the beginning of my research into one of mankind's most disfiguring skin problems.

We were not successful in treating Mr. H. at that time. The only temporary benefit he received was derived from the sun-filled days of Colorado. He left the hospital knowing full well that the lesions would soon return as they had in the past.

Fifteen years elapsed before I contacted Mr. H. again, for by then I had successfully treated several psoriasis cases. While our reunion was joyous, I was shocked by his appearance. He was a mere shadow of his former self, looking gaunt and tired and decidedly underweight. The spring to his step was gone. Every movement was slow and deliberate, and his speech was that of a man who had been "through the mill." Five years earlier he had suffered a massive heart attack and was hospitalized for several weeks with little hope of recovery. Miraculously, however, he pulled through, but only to lead a life bordering on invalidism.

He was still suffering with psoriasis. Upon examining him I found his lesions to be just as extensive and severe as ever. I showed him before and after photographs of my patients, and he expressed particular interest when I explained the significant role played by diet in alleviating psoriasis, which we were unaware of fifteen years ago. The story he then told me lent credence to the entire theory.

During his hospital stay he was fed intravenously for several weeks. During this period, a miracle seemed to take place; his psoriasis completely disappeared! The doctors had no explanation, and he was equally amazed. Not even a trace of the lesions remained, and since no one knew the reason for this unusual occurrence, it was simply considered "extraordinary"—and forgotten.

He related that upon being discharged from the hospital he was still perfectly clear of any lesions and went home to his "normal" diet. In no time at all, the psoriasis returned with a vengeance.

"What is your 'normal' diet?" I asked. "Rare roast beef and tomatoes," he replied. "I eat tomatoes by the bushel!"

Unfortunately, it will never be known whether or not Mr. H. could have benefited by my regimen, for he died shortly after my visit of an apparent second heart attack.

The fact is that for the relatively short period of time he was fed intravenously, he did not eat two of the major restricted items of the diet, red beef and tomatoes. This allowed his body time to detoxify. As a result, the lesions disappeared.

I contend that in severe cases of psoriasis, a medically supervised period of intravenous feeding could accelerate the detoxification process. This, however, is for medical authorities to decide. An experience such as that of Mr. H., as well as those reported by other patients, in my opinion, seems to justify further empirical studies. Techniques for detoxifying the body, such as intravenous feeding, may well be looked upon someday as a primary therapy in itself for many diseases.

Truth Is Where You Find It

In September, 1979, I gave a psoriasis lecture during an A.R.E. conference. As most speakers know, if their talk is well received, there is usually a gathering of people around them from the audience when the presentation is over, ready to ask more questions. I enjoy their additional inquiries and welcome them. They have a chance to learn more—and so do I.

After this particular lecture, a woman in the audience came up to me and said, "Doctor, I have something to tell you about psoriasis." To which I quickly responded, "Please do."

"Well," she continued, "my former husband had psoriasis all over his body for several years. At the same time, I was suffering from migraine headaches. We went to all kinds of doctors for many years for our respective problems, without results. Then, for reasons unrelated to our health problems, we divorced. Within a month, his psoriasis cleared up and my migraine headaches disappeared."

Now, I certainly do not advocate divorce in order to rid oneself of psoriasis—but, in this particular case, it seemed to have been the answer.

On the other side of the coin, however, there is the story of J.R., a beautiful young lady and patient of mine with a most severe case of psoriasis that she had been suffering with since childhood. She came from a family as beautiful as she was. Love radiated in the home which lent the needed support she had to have all her life. Yet, she was so severely afflicted that she thought she could never consider marrying and raising a family.

It took six months of complete dedication to the regimen for the changes to take place. At the end of that time, her condition was so greatly improved that the idea of marrying no longer seemed remote. Shortly thereafter, she married a very fine man who completely supported her endeavors to clear her skin of psoriasis. Today, this woman enjoys her husband, two children, and vibrant health. Since she now lives on the West Coast, she periodically informs me of her condition. At present (1990), she is—"just fine except for a little spot or two"—a far cry from being literally covered.

As important as every measure is in following the regimen, it cannot be overemphasized that cooperation and encouragement on the part of the person closest to the patient is absolutely vital.

Unhappy Mother's Day

Many fixations are so deeply rooted in our subconscious mind that the cause of a problem often evades us. An interesting case was that of a young girl (not my patient) who was completely cleared of psoriasis by a course of treatment I was not aware of, only to have it return in full bloom on Mother's Day. However, as the holiday passed, so did her psoriasis.

The patient herself provided a possible explanation. As a child, she became afflicted with psoriasis. In order to offset the psychological trauma brought about by this disease, her devoted mother gave her more love and attention than all her other children. As long as her mother was alive, this young girl had the emotional support she needed. After she died, however, that support system was gone. Because of this loss, her body reacted emotionally by breaking out in psoriatic lesions whenever Mother's Day came around.

To me, the above case indicates a return of toxicity to the body that was emotional in nature, demonstrating the incredible powers of the subconscious faculty within each and every one of us.

No Love—No Food—No Psoriasis!

In October of 1984, Miss L.W., a lovely nineteen year old girl, came into the office, a victim of psoriasis since the age of three. The problem was primarily confined to the scalp. Eventually, however, it began to appear as "spots" across the shoulders, upper arms, the breast plate area, and abdomen.

As I interviewed her with her mother, she began to see the importance of diet for the first time. It was obvious that she had been eating all the wrong foods, particularly Italian, her favorite, with its sauces and spices, as well as "junk" food. I convinced her that this was a major cause of her problem. In retrospect she concurred, for during the summer of '84, a breakup with her boy friend of four years triggered a starvation strike. For a month, she did not eat any of her customary foods, but sustained herself with water and very light foods. The result was that her psoriasis cleared up almost 100%.

After she recovered from her emotional trauma, she began to revert back to her old eating habits and the psoriasis soon returned. Despite this, she did not connect the recurrence with her diet until I brought it to her attention.

Intravenous—Again!

Mr. E. L. had psoriasis for about two years. Due to unrelated causes, he also developed problems, congenital in nature, known as arterial-venal malformation (AVM). A rather extensive surgical procedure was begun requiring long-term hospitalization which included intravenous feeding for a considerable period of time. His psoriasis slowly cleared up— completely!

Again, as in the case of Mr. H., his doctors were as amazed as he was, but they offered no explanation. They were satisfied that the arterial-venal malformation was successfully resolved. Although pleased by the fact that his psoriasis cleared up simultaneously, they were not interested in investigating that area of his health. He was released. The psoriasis returned when he returned to his favorite foods: red meat, vinegar, peppers and tomatoes!

This was the second time a similar result followed intravenous feeding. The inference here is that it is not some mysterious substance within the intravenous solution that helped clear the skin, but a case of what *was not* entering his body in the form of acid-forming foods.

Effects of Shellfish

I relate a story of one of my patients that borders on being a classic account, as to whether or not shellfish plays such an important role in controlling psoriasis in some people.

Mrs. E.C. had one of the most severe cases of psoriasis I have ever encountered. This women had experienced virtually every known form of therapy over a 25 year period. What little improvement took place was always short-lived. She came to my office on March 13, 1985.

After the usual indoctrination, Mrs. E.C. embarked on the regimen and, although painstakingly tedious, it was not too long before she felt the beneficial effects of the new approach. I made it quite clear that it might take a year or more of constant adherence to the regimen. She agreed. Improvement was slow but steady. She felt generally better, the scaling lessened, and the success of her efforts was clearly visible to her and her fellow employees.

As is often the case, she had to experiment for herself. She had to be convinced that diet played such an important role. She called on July 31, 1985, to inform me of how great she was doing until... "I had a *few* crabs, Dr. Pagano, and the next day my back just broke out so bad that I can't believe it. Now I am convinced I can't break the diet." I asked her what she meant by a "few" crabs. She answered, "Well, maybe eight or ten at one sitting." Eight or ten, I advised her, are not just a few. Probably, if she had eaten one or two crabs, her body could have handled it, but eight or ten caused an allergic reaction that blossomed into a violent attack. This, I told her, was "good" because she now knew that her system could not tolerate shellfish, at least not in the amount that she had eaten.

One of my cases, however, that of young B.M., indicates that with some people, even a small amount of shellfish is enough to cause a reaction. After this young lady was completely clear of guttate psoriasis for two months, she ate one and one half crabs. Her mother related that, within three hours, her lesions began to appear on her face, knees, and elbows. She immediately went on the raw apple diet and had an enema. The psoriasis began to clear overnight. A week before school started, her skin broke out again. Saffron tea fumes on the face and castor oil packs over the abdomen, particularly the right side, and Epsom Salts baths, quickly brought it under control. It is now almost two years since she responded so favorably and has remained clear ever since.

As in the previous case of E.C., she no longer has to prove to herself that diet plays such an important role in controlling psoriasis. They both know that they have only themselves to blame if their problem returns.

The Effect of Wearing Synthetic Fabrics

As mentioned in my previous chapter on eczema, the fact is that patients who wear nylon or synthetic garments sometimes have an adverse reaction to this material, especially after their skin has been cleared up. One patient, after doing exceptionally well, came back with her entire torso inflamed. It looked as though the healing process had reversed itself. Upon close inspection and questioning, however, we discovered a perfect outline on her body that followed the contour of her bathing suit. Just prior to this flare-up, the patient revealed that she had worn a nylon bathing suit. This reaction had been observed before when another patient also wore nylon or synthetic leotards. The line of demarcation could easily be noted. Because skin cannot breathe properly under synthetics, I concluded that these fabrics, in fact, caused this adverse reaction. Consequently, my advice then was to wear only cotton undergarments and bathing suits containing as little synthetic fiber as possible, preferably consisting mainly of cotton. Since making this observation, my suggestion proved to be quite beneficial to this patient as well as several others.

Using Vitamin E

Although Vitamin E was not mentioned earlier relative to psoriasis, one patient tried rubbing it into heavily scaled areas, using the liquid and/or cream form and achieved encouraging results.

The patient explained that Cuticura ointment did loosen the scales, but that the Vitamin E did not need to be worked in so vigorously. It removed the scales more quickly and the lesions broke up faster. She only used the Vitamin E cream (5000 i.u.) and no longer had to sleep with the oils and ointments. This substance tends to prevent thickening of the lesions, is easy to apply, relatively inexpensive and has little odor. Another advantage is that it also keeps the skin softer throughout the day. Similar results have often occurred by using Hydrophilic Ointment (See chapter "External Applications.")

If some natural measure is discovered that helps a psoriasis patient, the information is then passed on to other patients for them to utilize if they so choose. Time and space does not permit my going into all the interesting stories that have been observed when dealing with psoriasis. What is important, however, is to realize that there are many occasions when seemingly difficult problems have simple solutions. The aforementioned stories will undoubtedly relate to some patients who have had similar experiences.

Chapter 18

The Emotional Factor

Perhaps the most common question asked by psoriatics on their initial visit to the office is:

"Doctor, isn't psoriasis due to nerves?"

Answer: "Yes, it could be—but not always."

By "nerves" they do not mean the anatomical nerve connections to and from the spinal column, as previously described. What they mean by nerves in this case is nervous tension, irritability, aggravation, uptightness, domestic pressure of one kind or another; in other words, their feelings about things, their emotional state—the emotional factor.

Although one cannot *see* or measure emotions, one can certainly witness or experience their effects. In the case of psoriasis, it is these negative emotions that could start the chain reaction leading to hyperacidity in the system over an extended period of time which can contribute to an eventual breakdown of the intestinal walls.

Throughout the Cayce works we are constantly being reminded to curb our hostilities toward others. Not that we are ever to be a doormat, but to hold grudges and ill feelings toward others, even if apparently justified, only results in poisoning our own system. In fact, such attitudes can turn a body acidic even more readily than eating the wrong foods.

Chemical analysis of the perspiration of criminals has proven that the secretions of the body undergo certain distinct changes under the influence of different emotions. It is possible to trace the existence of hidden anger, fear, grief or remorse and distinguish one from the other, merely from this chemical difference in the fluids.

The perspiration of an angry man contains deadly poisons. More familiar are the facts that extreme fright or anger will poison or dry up the milk in the breasts of a nursing mother and even the lesser emotions of worry or annoyance will vitiate its quality. Violent grief or terror will so affect the coloring matter of the glands at the roots of the hair as to turn the hair white in a few hours. Good news brightens the eyes and straightens the stooping figure; bad news blanches the cheek and destroys the appetite; and confirmed invalids have many times found undreamed of strength when obliged to meet some great emergency unaided.

Virgil said of his soldiers, "They are able because they *think* they are able," and Mulford's theory that the quality of thought determines the body's condition is well founded. This is no less true in nervous ailments than in others, but in these it is more quickly and easily proven because of the close, direct relation between the brain and nervous system.

The term neurodermatitis was coined in the year 1891 by two French physicians, Louis Brocq and Leonard Jacquet, to describe skin disorders that have their origin in emotional states. In the same year, a Russian scientist by the name of A. G. Polotchoff, suggested that emotional upsets were sometimes among the causes of psoriasis.

Since then, research, especially by psychologically oriented dermatologists, has established that skin disorders often cause psychological problems, and vice-versa.

One of my patients definitely traces the origin of his psoriasis to a painful divorce he experienced twenty years ago, even though he is happily married now. With another, her psoriasis considerably improved after she married "Mr. Right;" with another, her psoriasis cleared when she was divorced.

What does all this tell us? It tells us, loud and clear, that *our personal reaction to a situation determines the effect that particular situation has upon us.*

Jane E. Brody, in her well-documented article, "Emotions Found to Influence Nearly Every Human Ailment" (New York Times, Tuesday, May 24, 1983), refers to the work of Dr. George F. Solomon, a University of California psychiatrist:

"Mind and body are inseparable," he said. "The brain influences all sorts of physiological processes that were once thought not to be centrally regulated."

"The studies also show that the traditional concept of 'stress' as a demanding life event is too imprecise to use as a measurement of how stress affects health. What is distressing to one person may be stimulating to another. Rather, the researchers are finding it is how a person responds to life events, not the events themselves, that influences susceptibility to disease. The studies indicate that failure to cope well with stress can impair a person's ability to fight off illness; whereas, adequate coping with a high-stress life may reflect 'psychological hardiness' that is actually protective." (Reprinted by permission.)

That we have within ourselves the power to *decide* our reaction to life's events is to me one of the most profound discoveries of our time, for it places our state of happiness (or misery) largely in our own hands.

For instance, to be slighted, insulted or purposefully abused is to conjure up the most basic of human emotions, anger. Yet, uncontrolled anger has caused pain and hardship to evolve by its accompanying state of hatred and resentment. The original cause, whether by hurtful words or acts, is often lost, forgotten, or seen as inconsequential compared to the stormy aftermath.

Can any of us in America forget the alleged gasoline crisis that took place in the winter of 1973? Lines of cars edged in front of each other, triggering violent tempers, physical harm and even murder. Because of the hatred that ensued, mental poisons took over the minds of many motorists which resulted in penalties with which many are still paying the price in the form of legal fees, physical injuries and/or jail sentences.

Why did all this occur? Because of negative emotional states. Fortunately, the above illustrations are extremely rare. It is the every day, relatively minor irritations that we must guard against. This does not mean we should become passive, impotent, slothful personalities.

No one is asked or expected to be abused by anyone. To express oneself, even forcefully, is in keeping with sound mental health. The trick is not to carry inner resentments and condemnatory thoughts. To reiterate, it can poison the blood even faster than eating the wrong food.

Make no mistake about it—the one who hates suffers internally more than the one who is hated. For one thing, the one who is hated may never be aware of it, which is quite often the case. But the one who does the hating is certainly aware of it day by day and experiences within himself the aftereffects hate carries—an internal build-up of poisons, toxins and acidity.

It was my pleasure and honor to personally meet one of the most renowned thinkers of our age, Manly Palmer Hall, while I was an intern in Denver, Colorado. His inspirational words from "Healing, The Divine Art," ring out on this subject as clearly today as they did then.

"The Negative Emotion of Fear— Fear Fixations and Phobias

Another irrational emotion is hatred; defined as an intense form of dislike, it is far more dangerous to the one who hates than to the object of the hatred."[1]

"No Health Where Hate Is— Hatred, The Irrational Emotion

No one can hate and be healthy at the same time. It is essentially human for a person to dislike those who have injured him, filched his worldly goods, or frustrated his reasonable accomplishments. The other person's fault may be great, but the one who hates him, no matter how just the cause, has the fault which is the greater. The Scriptural admonition, to do good to those who despitefully use us, is not only a noble statement of spiritual truth, but a cardinal tenet of psychotherapy."[2]

Conversely, the one who practices patience, gentleness and kindness tends to experience within himself the aftereffects of such attitudes: radiant health, cheerfulness and joy. The triune principle of Mind, Body and Spirit cannot be separated. Practice keeping the mind pure of prejudice, hates and jealousies, and the body responds with increased energy, vigor and vitality. Keep the body cleansed internally and externally, flexible and active, and the mind reacts with enthusiasm, cheerfulness and acuity.

To the patient who justifies a negative attitude by saying, "But I can't help it, this is the way I am," I say, "Have you tried?" Did any of us know how to ride a bicycle when we were youngsters before taking the necessary falls and lumps? Were we all born swimmers? No, we had to learn everything. The same applies to thinking processes as they do to sports or to any other physical or mental activity. Learn to think in a way that would serve your best interests as far as your reaction is concerned. A different viewpoint may be all that's necessary. It is a known fact that the heat of a violent argument can be offset instantaneously by exercising a sense of humor. I can recall a true story of how a little old lady warded off "a would-be mugger" who confronted her on a dark street, gun in hand, with full intentions of robbing her of what little she had and possibly causing physical harm. When he jumped in front of her with his gun pointing at her face and demanding her purse, she responded with, "Oh, young man, what is the trouble? Can't you find a job? You know I don't blame you, finding a job is so hard these days. Is that a real gun? May I see it? I never saw a real one before." His answer was "Damn it lady, you got me all confused." He ran off into the night.

She did not respond the way he anticipated. Panic, fear and submission would have been the "normal" reaction. But, confusion claimed the mind of the perpetrator because her reaction broke all the rules. By her calm, serene attitude, she avoided being robbed, harmed, possibly shot, while at the same time, preventing him from committing a crime, at least in this case.

The idea brought forth here is to realize that we have, to a very large extent, the power to control *our reaction* to whatever happens to us. To put it more succinctly: It is not what happens to us, it is what *we think of* what happens to us that determines our misery or happiness.

Our Built-In Antenna

The idea that aggravating circumstances, or one's reaction to the circumstance, have a decided effect on the skin is nothing new to most psoriatics. One of my patients in particular has no problem relating to that concept. Afflicted for twenty years, he readily admits to experiencing all sorts of sensations on his skin, usually with job-related pressures. His skin practically screams at him when he is upset. Itching and tingling, blotching and flare-ups are the immediate reaction. Although he follows all the rules from a dietary point of view, here is a case where we both agree that his basic cause is emotional.

In an exceptionally informative article entitled, "Bringing Peace to Embattled Skin," (Psychology Today—Feb. 1982) by Ted A. Grossbart,

Ph.D.,* clinical psychologist at Beth Israel Hospital in Boston and in the Department of Psychiatry at Harvard Medical School, states:

> "The causes of skin disorders are varied. Heredity plays a role in some. Bacteria, viruses and physical and chemical irritants are important in others. Whatever the underlying cause, emotional problems may increase the frequency and severity of attacks. They may even be the fundamental cause of some disorders." [3]

He continues with:

> "The skin lives an emotional life of its own. It remembers, rages, cries and punishes for real or imagined sins."[4]

There is no question that we are dealing with a two-edged sword. The condition of the skin effects the emotions, and the emotions effect the skin. There is an interaction between the two that cannot be denied.

Fortunately, helping one often helps the other which perhaps explains why we should try to keep our thoughts constructive. When the patient learns to control the emotions, the skin improves. When external applications help the skin, the emotions are decidedly affected by a more joyful, hopeful countenance. This is why I do not discourage patients, particularly those severely affected, to incorporate controlled ultraviolet light or other proven medical procedures to help clear the skin if they so desire. It would not interfere with the regimen. If it helps the patient feel better about himself, it is a plus. It is best, however, that my patients continue with all the other measures as outlined. If and when UV light or some such therapy temporarily helps clear the skin, I emphasize that they should not be lulled into believing the problem is permanently resolved and that they can now safely discard the regimen.

At Times, A Paradox!

There are patients who, from all outward appearances, want to rid themselves of the disease; but when success is forthcoming, they retract, break the rules and *allow* the disease to return. They, themselves,

*Ted A. Grossbart, Ph.D. has co-authored the book SKIN DEEP: A Mind/Body Program for Healthy Skin with Carl Sherman, Ph.D., New York: William Morrow, 1986.

undoubtedly deny playing such a game. Nevertheless, in some cases, it is true. For years they may have been the center of attention with sympathy and pity constantly showered upon them because of their dilemma. They *subconsciously* feel that ridding themselves of the disease is a threat to being the center of attention. They are in a mental quandary. On the one hand they want to be cured; on the other, they fear they will lose that prize we all desire—attention. When they come to grips with this paradox and see it for what it is, they usually improve.

Moreover, having the disease has become such a habit that some patients cannot *visualize* themselves without it. But they must, or the results would be slight, if at all. They must get rid of the "old friend" as they would an "old sore."

There are those who also feel they must retain the disease as a form of self-punishment for reasons only they know. Whether or not they deserve such punishment is beside the point. The fact is they *think* they do, so they become their own judge and jury. To such personalities I try to get across to be less harsh on themselves, take life easier and try to "count your blessings instead of sheep" as Irving Berlin melodically advised.

A Different Twist

Stressful situations are usually linked to negative circumstances. We often connect ulcers, headache, nervousness and conditions such as indigestion to an unhappy situation. Perhaps it is our working conditions, a love affair that has gone sour, poor family harmony or school pressures. We must also recognize the fact that stressful feelings can come from joyful occasions that may also have a deleterious effect upon the person involved, depending on his or her attitude. For instance, one patient was doing extremely well with her psoriatic arthritic condition when suddenly there was a flare-up of the arthritis in her joints, although her skin remained clear. We went over all aspects of the regimen to see if she was inadvertently violating parts of the principles of treatment. She was not. It came out later in the conversation that she had just become engaged to be married a few days before the flare-up occurred. When I asked if she thought this placed her under an emotional strain, even though it was a joyous occasion, she quickly nodded yes. This was the only explanation we could come up with and she fully appreciated its implication.

At first glance the above may seem to be a contradiction in terms, but I assure you it is not. You see, it was not the joyous occasion that triggered her arthritis, but the *worry* that accompanied the event, even though happiness underlies the whole situation.

Again, let us be mindful that it is not the emotional experience that determines our physical reaction, it is our *attitude* toward the occurrence that directs our response.

The Mind Worketh Miracles—Or Misery!

I often recall a conversation I had with a patient while at the hospital in Denver. It closely parallels this type of reaction but to a much more devastating degree. This gentleman had been working at Montgomery Ward for several years. His goal was to become a department manager. He strove for it in every way possible for many years. Then the day arrived. He was notified that as of a certain date he would take over the entire department as manager. The next morning he could not get out of bed. A spastic form of hysterical paralysis crippled his entire body. It was subsequently diagnosed as spastic multiple sclerosis. It was a progressive disease with no hope for a cure.

Here is a situation where a man was advanced to the position he wanted, strove for and apparently desired but, in his case, much to his dismay and for reasons that may never be known, his physical reaction resulted in a severe illness. Was it because of a subconscious fear of what the new job entailed? To someone else, the reaction would be different, but to him it was obviously more than he could bear. Perhaps it was the final straw that triggered off an underlying disease process already in the making. We will never know for the patient did not survive.

On The Brighter Side

For approximately two years it was my good fortune to have as my evening secretary a most delightful young lady whom we will call "Judy." A most attractive, friendly and energetic girl of 18, Judy held three jobs at one time while attending school and was quite popular in her circle of friends. She had a problem, though—psoriasis.

It was her older sister who had started coming to me for psoriasis with complete satisfactory results after eighteen months. Judy had developed blotches, particularly on her legs and waist area. One day, she came in with the psoriatic blotches all over her lovely face. An immediate regimen of cleansing was adhered to and in a relatively short time, with concentrated use of Saffron Tea and enemas or colonics, she cleared up nicely. Then the blotches would pop up again for no apparent reason.

The end of the school year arrived, and Judy decided to spend the summer out West on a ranch as a waitress. She sent several resumes out and finally decided on a beautiful dude ranch in northern Colorado. It would be her first time away from home, which was on the east coast. Needless to say, she had the normal feeling of anxiety, knowing she would be on her own for the first time, in a strange place, with new faces, thousands of miles from home.

At the appointed time, Judy left for Colorado in her little car with a few pieces of luggage, her cowboy hat and—her psoriasis.

Reports from her family all indicated she loved Colorado. A letter to me proved to verify she had found a new life in that beautiful land. She was very popular and efficient in her job. The owners loved her and wished her to "stay on" all winter which she decided to do.

In early September, I planned a vacation in Wyoming with the thought that I may be able to stop at the ranch where Judy worked and surprise her. Well, I did surprise her, but not half as much as she surprised me.

After our emotional greeting at the ranch and hours of stories of her great experiences expressing her enthusiasm for her work and the land, she spoke of her *former* problem of psoriasis. I was amazed to see that there wasn't a mark on her. She related that she did take the Saffron Tea and Slippery Elm "fairly" regularly but was not, and could not be, totally strict with the diet.

When I asked about the reason for such a dramatic result, she answered without the slightest doubt, "It's my contentment." She was so inwardly happy with the conditions and her environment that she no longer produced her own poisons due to "up tight" feelings at home.

Was it her parents that caused this strained feeling? Hardly. Judy was trying to get them to move out West as well, which they seriously contemplated.

Obviously, I do not recommend that patients pick up stakes and change residence to rid themselves of psoriasis. This, however, is what happened in Judy's case. Each patient may have an entirely different cause. The goal is to seek out the cause of the particular condition and do everything that is possible to change it.

Yes, contentment played a large part in Judy's success, but so did nutritious food on the ranch's regular meal schedule. In a letter to me, she stated the following:

"Eating three square meals a day made a big difference in my elim-inating process. Regular, scheduled, balanced meals lead to a bowel movement once a day instead of maybe one every two or three days. This, I believe, played a big part in the disappearance of my psoriasis. Besides being a happier, more energetic person (good diet played a big part in this), I was eating regularly more nutritiously than I had my whole life."

So here we have a change of dietary habits, emotional contentment and beautiful surroundings. It all contributed to Judy's victory over psori-asis. To this day, she remains clear.

A Triune Comparison

When one takes the time to examine the teachings of three giants in their respective fields and find that they come to the same conclusion on the effect joy or anger has on the human organism, I, for one, would want to pay attention, listen and learn.

Compare The Following:

Pottenger—(Scientific):

"Such emotions as fear, anger, and pain, act upon the sympathet-ics as shown by Cannon and his coworkers, while joy and happi-ness tend to preserve the normal physiologic nervous and endocrine equilibrium."[5]

Manly P. Hall—(Philosophic):

"Harmony in the mind results in the increasing health of the body; and harmony in the body improves the disposition of the mind."[6]

Edgar Cayce—(Spiritual):

"Anger causes poisons to be secreted by the glands (Adrenals prin-cipally). Joy has the opposite effect." (All the glands are involved to some extent.)[7]

Can it be any clearer? It should answer the question on whether or not man should engage in "the pursuit of happiness." My belief is he should indeed, for then and only then, is he living in his natural state. It should come as no surprise to him, however, if he finds his "pursuit" originates and terminates within his own self.

What You "See" Is What You Get

Can the mind have such an effect as to create a skin reaction by either actual or imaginary irritants? It most certainly can. An eye opening incident took place when two Japanese physicians, Y. Ikemi and S. A. Nakagawa, experimented with a plant similar to poison ivy. Placing a patient under hypnosis, they applied the poison leaf to the skin with the added suggestion that it was harmless. There was no skin reaction. Conversely, if a leaf that was harmless was placed on the skin with the suggestion that it was toxic, a decided reaction took place. The patient's skin became red and irritated. The subconscious mind of the patient did not argue the point. It accepted the suggestion as truth and reacted accordingly. More on this score was covered in my chapter, "Right Thinking." For now, suffice it to say that the mind, through thought or emotion, can and does affect skin reactions.

A Possible Solution

The causes of our emotional makeup are not always obvious. They could be so deep-rooted within our subconscious that only long, arduous self-analysis or professional help may provide some answers.

My personal conclusion, based on a lifetime of observing "successful" personalities versus the "losers" is that the answer lies largely in the vision we have of *ourselves*. Do you like what you see in the mirror? If you don't, you have another job to do other than clear your skin—you must *start today* to appreciate yourself in a healthy, divinely inspired way, not as one on an ego trip. This means to like the kind of person you are and be at peace with your inner self.

What if you don't like the kind of person you are? Then start doing something that will help you like the person you are—DO SOMETHING FOR SOMEBODY ELSE.

Throughout the ages of man, the most frequent advice regarding physical and mental health is to adopt the attitude of helping others. Depending on your attitude, this is not all that difficult. It does not require earth-shattering demonstrations. All it takes is being kind and gentle, just being patient, *first* with yourself, then with others.

It is the everyday little things, common to all of us, that makes for the realization of this *principle*. We all can't be an Albert Schweitzer serving the sick and depressed in the wilds of Africa or a Mother Teresa administering to the needy through the slums of Calcutta. For one thing, theirs was an inspirationally guided mission that came from the very depths of their souls. Unless this same inner guidance does the directing, the end result would be pure mimicry and probably end in dismal failure. No, it is the world around us, our family, neighbors, friends, associates where those little kindnesses have their meaning.

The Day of the Cookie

One day, a few years ago, I could not help but experience this feeling of self-worth by an unexpected simple act I committed while returning from a house call. While walking to my car in a depressed, poverty-ridden area of a neighboring town, I passed a bakery shop and was magnetically drawn back to it by the aroma of fine baking that permeated the air. With my nose and hand pressed against the windowpane admiring the array of cookies being placed on display, I confronted myself with advice that they were fattening and probably not good for me. The argument lasted about two seconds. In three seconds, I found myself ordering five dollars worth of those fine, healthy, delicious cookies.

I hurried out, box of cookies in hand, in a rush to satisfy my gluttonous appetite. The minute I stepped through the door, I glanced down and saw a little tot of a girl right where I had been standing a few minutes before. Her nose was pressed against the window with both hands flat against the pane. She was feasting her eyes on the same cookie display. I stopped for a moment, then continued toward my car. Somehow my steps toward the car were getting slower and slower. I never made it to the car. Turning quickly, I walked back to the little girl, found her still pressed against the window, got her attention and said, handing her the cookies, "Here little girl, these are for you and your family."

The look of total shock lit up her face as she cautiously took the box of cookies, looked at me and hurried off—to her father, who was parked halfway down the street in his brand new 450 SL Mercedes! Slowly I turned and walked to my eight-year old Pontiac, got behind the wheel, managed to get it started, and drove off.

By the time I reached my office, I got over the feeling of being a total blithering idiot. In time, however, after giving it further thought, I realized that it was my *intention* that really mattered and not my embarrassment. I helped brighten the little girl's day, and I felt good about myself. That feeling remained all day.

This, I believe, is what is meant by the "little things" that determine our self-worth. Besides, I concluded—so the father had a Mercedes. Who knows? Maybe the kid never had a cookie!

Helping Yourself and Others At The Same Time

Is there something we can do on a daily basis that can in some way be a blessing to ourselves and to those around us? Yes, there is, the simplicity of which is the reason it often evades us...SMILE!

There's an old philosophy that has weathered the test of time..."*to become, act as if.*" It means if you want to be happy, act as if you are happy and in ways beyond knowing, the *spirit* of happiness will find its way into your soul and heart. Like anything else, it takes practice, but in time, the technique will pay off and you will find it works in many areas of life if given a chance.

One of the best methods of feeling a glow of happiness within is to smile, "even if it takes the hide off," as Cayce says.

Have you ever noticed how people in general just seem to migrate to the person who smiles? Why? Because I believe people who smile project an image of a person who is above it all. Did you ever see a President of the United States who didn't smile?—Especially in recent years? It indicates an inner strength, their feathers are not easily ruffled, they have a sense of humor toward life, and people subconsciously want that attitude to rub off on them.

I can attest to this when I personally had the honor of meeting H.H. The Dalai Lama after my talk on psoriasis in Bangalore, India. His pleasing countenance was contagious—he was always smiling. He came to America in 1990, after receiving the Nobel Peace Prize and, in an interview, emphasized the importance of smiling. He is a prime example of practicing what he preaches.

James Allen, in his classic, "As A Man Thinketh," observes:

> "Who does not love a tranquil heart, a sweet-tempered, balanced disposition? It does not matter whether it rains or shines, or what changes come to those possessing these blessings, for they are always sweet, serene and calm"[8]

On several speaking engagements, I often close with a poem that I feel is quite apropos to the principle of developing a constructive, cheerful countenance. On one particular occasion, while speaking before an A.R.E. regional conference in Philadelphia, I chose another ending for fear of being repetitious. I was somewhat surprised when the chairperson of the conference called me back to repeat the poem she heard me recite two years earlier. Others in the audience also expressed their desire to hear it again.

I close this chapter with that same little poem, *The Power of a Smile*, author unknown, for its impact on our awareness may very well be a key to a healthy, balanced emotional life.

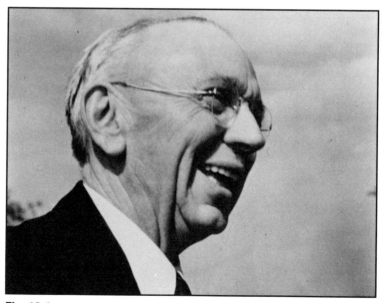

Fig. 18-1
The captivating smile of *Edgar Cayce*

The Power of a Smile

"YOU DON'T HAVE TO TELL
HOW YOU LIVE EACH DAY;
YOU DON'T HAVE TO TELL
IF YOU WORK OR PLAY.

A TRIED, TRUE BAROMETER
SERVES IN ITS PLACE.
HOWEVER YOU LIVE,
IT WILL SHOW IN YOUR FACE.

THE FALSENESS OR GOODNESS
YOU BEAR IN YOUR HEART
WILL NOT STAY INSIDE
WHERE IT FIRST GOT ITS START.

FOR SINEW AND BLOOD
ARE A THIN VEIL OF LACE:
WHAT YOU WEAR IN YOUR HEART
YOU WEAR ON YOUR FACE.

IF YOUR LIFE IS UNSELFISH,
IF FOR OTHERS YOU LIVE
FOR NOT WHAT YOU GET,
BUT HOW MUCH YOU GIVE;

IF YOU LIVE CLOSE TO GOD
IN HIS INFINITE GRACE,
YOU DON'T HAVE TO TELL IT,
IT SHOWS IN YOUR FACE."

REFERENCES

(Chapter 18—The Emotional Factor)

1. Manly P. Hall, *Healing, The Divine Art* (©1943 by Manly Palmer Hall, Los Angeles, California, Pub. by the Philosophical Research Society, Inc.) P. 260. (Reprinted by permission).
2. Ibid., p. 261.
3. Ted A. Grossbart, Ph.D., "Bringing Peace to Embattled Skin," *Psychology Today*, (Feb. 1982), p. 55. (Reprinted by permission).
4. Ibid., p. 59.
5. Francis Marion Pottenger, *Symptoms of Visceral Disease*, ed. 7, (St. Louis, 1953, The C.V. Mosby Co.), p. 135.
6. Manly P. Hall, p. 238.
7. Reading 281-54—The Edgar Cayce Readings, Association for Research and Enlightenment (A.R.E.), Virginia Beach, Virginia.
8. James Allen, *As A Man Thinketh*, (Mt. Vernon, NY, The Peter Pauper Press), pp. 58-59.

Chapter 19

What About The Failures?

To insinuate or even imply that I have always succeeded with a patient would not only be a gross exaggeration; it would be an inexcusable lie.

Certainly there have been failures—some are easily explained, others are not. The reasons remain evasive if the focus is placed only on the regimen and not on the patient as well. The question is—what caused the failure? Did the therapy fail, or did the patient (and doctor) fail the therapy? Until this question is honestly answered, one cannot judge if the regimen really does or does not work on a specific individual.

This I can say unequivocally: if the patient is sincere, follows through faithfully, allows adequate time for the procedure to work and is willing to change his lifestyle—particularly, his eating habits—then the chances of success are greatly enhanced.

Just by the law of averages, however, there is a certain percentage of people who will not respond to this or any other therapy, even if they follow it to the letter. It's anybody's guess why this occurs. Allowing for this unexplained percentage of failure, there is one common cause ascribed to most failures; *they stopped following the regimen.*

At times, the reasoning was quite clear—results were not fast enough. With others, desire for alcoholic drinks, sweets or rich foods overpowered their desire to clear the skin. And there were those who simply did not have a severe enough case to follow the discipline, especially the diet. All in all, even with these "unsuccessful" cases, some degree of improvement was shown with most of them. "Persistence" is the key word in the treatment of psoriasis, as it is in all successful endeavors.

"Advice" From the Uninformed

Another problem the patient as well as the physician must guard against are discouraging thoughts and comments from well-meaning, but uninformed relatives and friends. This is why I insist that a new patient bring a close relative or friend to the initial consultation. There is nothing like evidence, a track record of successful cases, and knowledge of the entire procedure that will convert a concerned friend into a helping hand to the patient. There have been countless times when the patient came alone for the initial interview, left the office encouraged and filled with enthusiasm, only to be discouraged by people who took neither the time nor the interest to investigate the process for themselves. The psoriatic doesn't need this type of influence. At times, it might be better for the patient not to say anything, proceed with the regimen and later, if successful, reveal the source of his or her accomplishment.

One effective method of showing results to the non-psoriatic as well as the psoriatic is the videotape, *Project: Psoriasis*—Part I and Part II. This film, in VHS playback format, shows results obtained over ten years, including interviews with patients seven to ten years after they were cleared. New patients can borrow the tape so that others will understand the regimen more thoroughly, see the results and feel justified in giving it a chance. So far, the reaction to it has been very positive. Once the facts are viewed, one is not so quick to condemn.

A Prime Example

Only the strong, positive attitude of one of my patients, Mrs. I.A., helped rid her body of psoriasis in three months after suffering with it for fifty years. She was bombarded on all sides by disparaging thoughts from her entire family when therapy began. Surely, a lesser person would have buckled under the strain. Here, however, was a dynamo. She was determined to succeed, and that positive thought carried her across the finish line. When she reached her objective, the same relatives who discouraged her admitted, "Well, maybe you did do the right thing after all!"

Not all people are blessed with the strong resolve of Mrs. I.A. They *need* encouragement, attention and love on the part of those around them in order to be successful. In cases of psoriasis, affection and interest shown by those closest to them, usually hasten the desired results, making the goal easier to attain and more complete.

Naturally, no one wishes to be diseased any longer than necessary, especially with something so miserable as psoriasis. The disease did not develop overnight. Therefore, it follows that it cannot be eliminated overnight. Here is where encouragement comes in.

Part of the physician's responsibility, as well as that of relatives and friends, is to constantly provide the patient with that encouragement in order to strengthen their resolve to get well. Arranging personal introductions between successful patients and new ones is one of the most valuable steps the doctor can take to further promote confidence and assurance.

It takes *time* to get sick, especially with a systemic type disease. Although logical, it is sometimes hard for a patient to grasp that it will also take time to get well. If the condition is not irreversible, however, and the proper measures are employed, it is amazing how quickly the body will bring itself into equilibrium. This point is stressed with new patients as much as are diet and other elements of the regimen.

A Most Irritating Problem

There is nothing more aggravating, frustrating, and mind-boggling than seeing some people struggle for the slightest improvement while others clear up in practically no time at all. Patience is a virtue and no researcher should be without it, but in all honesty, this is one of the most irritating problems I had to face in caring for a psoriasis patient.

There have been countless times when I was ready to throw in the towel and go on to newer and more promising things, when all at once a severe case would quickly clear up. This would encourage me until my newly found energy and enthusiasm was thwarted by new failures. I often asked myself why this happened. If this process is real and the principles are followed faithfully, shouldn't the right results *always* be attained?

I believe the answer lies, for one reason or another, within the patients themselves, and the successful cases are really the forerunners for further research. I have always maintained that if you want to be successful, you should do what successful people do. Although I prefer to concentrate on those who succeed, there is, however, a certain amount of comfort in observing the failures, for therein you may find a clue as to which direction to avoid.

Thomas A. Edison, American inventor of thousands of vitally useful products, advocated the value of failure—but only as a catalyst to persist until the answer was found. He must have done something right, for in his eighty-four years, (1847-1931) Thomas Alva Edison took out 1,093 patents, the most ever granted to any one person. As the practical-minded giver of light, Edison became the American Prometheus, the prophet of technological progress. With all the "failures" he experienced, the gems that he eventually brought forth prompted Congress in 1923 to put the "Value of Edison's Genius" at fifteen billion dollars. When asked what he would request from Aladdin's genie if he had the chance, he answered without hesitation, "My health!"[1]

Something, therefore, indeed can be said for failure; provided, however, it acts as a stimulus to continue to plod ahead, determined to find an answer. The question in my mind is no longer whether, if followed, the procedures contained herein work or not. The proverbial question now is, "Why does it work on some but not on others?" I postulate that if it works on *one* it has the *potential* to work on all. With this in mind, the ability of the practitioner to recognize each and every patient as an individual entity is primary in their case management. One must follow the principles practiced by the patients with a successful outcome. The cardinal rule, however, is to *tailor these principles to meet the needs of each patient.*

Reasons For Failure:

There are causes for failures as well as successes. To repeat the question—if many people completely succeed with this regimen, why do others fail? The most common reasons for the failure, according to my observations are the following:

1. Inability or lack of determination on the part of the patient to follow through long enough.

2. Discouragement on the part of relatives, friends and physicians unacquainted with this manner of therapy.

3. Lack of cooperation by the patient's spouse or guardian in preparing the proper foods outlined.

4. "X" the unknown. There are always failures that defy explanation. We have had our share, but fortunately, this number represents a small minority.

Do What Successful People Do

As mentioned earlier, I subscribe to the philosophy that if you want to be successful, study the lives of successful people.

Those patients who have succeeded followed every measure to the best of their ability and placed "getting well" uppermost in their mind. For instance, it never mattered to them what friends might say at a cocktail party when they drank ice water or seltzer with lime on the rocks instead of a highball. They took the time to study a menu while dining out and chose only permitted foods. They prepared their herb teas each day, took their Epsom Salts baths, and had spinal adjustments as recommended. They were guided by the philosophy, "Keep-on, Keeping-on!" until the desired results were attained.

Sweets and Alcohol

Two items seem to be the most difficult for a patient to give up or at least greatly curtail—sweets and alcohol. Excessive smoking is not far behind.

Candy is the leading culprit among sweets. Hard alcohol (gin, whiskey, vodka) or excessive quantities of beer is the problem with drinkers. In truth, many patients that I have encountered with either one or both of these addictions have a rather difficult time abstaining from them.

Fortunately, these cases are not the majority. Most patients do, in fact, place the clearing of their skin first. Those with the addiction, unless they learn to control their desires, face a lifetime of doctors, expense, and misery.

They Won't Believe It

One rather irritating attitude that fortunately is not encountered too often is to find patients refusing to admit or believe that it was this regimen that cleared them up after they had suffered for years with massive areas of lesions covering their bodies. One patient's girlfriend once called me secretly to tell me, "Doctor, I know it was the diet that completely cleared his skin, but he refuses to believe it. Now he went back to his old way of eating and he is covered again."

It was always puzzling to me why a patient would suddenly go off the diet knowing it could harm him or at least retard the cleansing process. I searched for a logical answer and, as is often the case, a successful psoriasis case came forth with an answer that made sense to me and to several other patients when I brought it to their attention.

It is because, as expressed by one particular patient, "You feel like you are in jail. You can't do this, you can't do that; you can't eat this, you can't eat that." Frustration sets in. But with one big difference—you can always open the door and walk out. A true prisoner does not have that option. When she opened the door and walked out, her psoriasis came back. It was then that she realized she did indeed have control over the situation. Once she overcame her "childish" attitude, as she put it, and followed the rules, she was free once again. Her skin cleared and remains as clear as she wants it to be.

Some patients attribute the results to exposure to the sun or ultraviolet treatments, but not the discipline of the dietary requirements and cleansing methods described herein. They are stymied, however, when I have them meet patients who completely cleared up *never* having exposed themselves to the sun or ultraviolet therapy of any kind.

I believe most of these patients feel secure by holding a negative view because that is their habitual way of thinking and they do not like changing their lifestyles, or giving up, even for a short time, their favorite food and drink. Then again, maybe they have been through so much from an orthodox treatment point of view that they refuse to believe the answer could be so simple.

It is not unusual for some patients with a severe degree of psoriasis to quit this regimen in "midstream" *even when results are beginning to become apparent*! Another frustrating experience for the doctor is when positive changes in the skin are seen and the patient admits to it, progress is confirmed by the spouse, only to find the patient goes back to his or her old lifestyle, knowing full well the lesions will return—and they do! It seems the patient simply wanted to test this procedure to see if it really worked. They seem to adopt the attitude, "OK, it works—so eventually I'll get around to it. In the meantime, I'll eat and drink what I want." When such incidents occur, and fortunately, they are infrequent, the reason is obvious—lack of discipline concerning diet. Such patients would like to rid themselves of psoriasis, but they consider the price too high. It is incredible what they will suffer, by inconvenience, embarrassment, or disfigurement in order to satisfy their dietary habits. Such patients are headed for difficult times, if they refuse to change within their heart and mind.

I have heard some patients who claim, "My psoriasis just went away and never came back." I have no reason to disbelieve that. But, such incidents are extremely rare. To those who wait for it to just go away, I say, *don't count on it*! Take the action steps to conquer the disease and stop being "childish" about it. Then and only then will they have control, if not a complete cure, of the disease.

"Intellectualizing"—A Pitfall?

Mr. H.M. had a severe case of psoriasis on his face (which is rather rare), his back, chest, and particularly his legs. He came to my office seeking any method to stop this progression which had started only six months earlier. He was a kind, well liked, cheerful, hard-working individual. Quite frankly, I wasn't convinced within myself that he would be successful because he wasn't "intellectual" enough about it. He didn't question the procedure. With the invaluable aid of his wife, he simply followed the instructions to the letter . Within three months, he was completely clear throughout his face, chest, back and most of his arms with some remaining lesions disappearing on his legs. Three months later, he was 100% clear. When I asked him, as I do all my successful cases, what he thought was the cause of his psoriasis—he quickly answered, "Junk food—you said stay away from it, so I did!"

The "intellectuals" who question everything, rather than practice the procedure called for, are still battling their skin problem. Mind you, I am not against the person who seeks answers to questions. I am annoyed by the person who seeks answers that fit their preconceived notions, and if the answers don't fit, dismisses them.

From *The Concurrence*, William Kearny Carr said it best:

"However much intellect is to be commended, it has its disadvantage, since it increases our doubts, and therefore becomes the greatest hindrance to our success. All progress is from below, upward; hence we should expect to hear wisdom from the humble and unintelligent. They have not their intellect trained so as to doubt, and hence they often see intuitively and instantly what so often comes laboriously, if at all, to the better disciplined intellect."

Therefore, if the patients will get out of their own way and sincerely seek answers, answers are provided.

At the risk of being repetitive to my readers, I must emphasize that the success of this or any other worthwhile accomplishment must have as its foundation the building blocks of *Patience and Persistence*. Without these two mental ingredients, the structure upon which this principle of healing is based will crumble into dust. This approach is the very opposite of so many psoriasis sufferers who are satisfied with a "quick fix." Until they view psoriasis as a systemic problem that must be managed systemically, successful results are hard, if not impossible, to attain. Once they "get on" to this overall picture of the problem, the approach they take to the disease takes on a new dimension and, if practiced faithfully, more often than not, brings about the desired end result.

REFERENCES

(Chapter 19—What About the Failures?)

1. Wyn Wachhorst, *Thomas Alva Edison—An American Myth*, (Cambridge, Mass. & London, England, The MIT Press, ©. 1981).

Chapter 20

The Question of Recurrence

The question of whether or not psoriasis will return after it clears is and should be of primary concern to the patient. Obviously, one would not look enthusiastically upon a mode of therapy that offered only fleeting results—yet, this is often the case in orthodox management.

There are only two reasons why psoriasis may return after it has been cleared: (1) The root cause of the disease remains, or (2) The patient returned to his or her old way of life too soon. Of the two, the latter is, from my observation, the major reason for the recurrence.

If the psoriasis clears by following this regimen in the first place, we can safely assume we have attacked the primary cause successfully. Therefore, if it returns, the only logical conclusion is that the patient reactivated the primary cause of the disease. What is the solution? Simple. Return to the basic regimen.

Although I mentioned this before, it deserves repetition. *Once patients clear their skin of psoriasis by following this regimen, they never fear the disease again!* That is not to say they will never break out again. They most certainly can and usually do, if they grossly abuse their diet in particular. The reason they no longer fear it is that they *know* how to control it on their own to a large extent. I have often observed patients on their first visit, gripped with apprehension visualizing themselves getting progressively worse, which may lead to periodic hospitalization throughout their lives, and possible invalidism. The whole scene changes, however, when they get well with not a mark on their bodies and confidently revert to some of their favorite eating habits with the attitude, "Well, if it pops out again, I'll just go on the diet." There is nothing wrong with that—as long as they never let it get out of hand again. This is how effective it has been for some patients. With others there seems to be *no* return at all regardless of how much they stray from the diet, but this is not usually the case.

I can only surmise with these apparent successful cases that they stayed on the regimen long enough to allow proper and effective healing of the thin intestinal walls. There is no question that they can now live with it, or shall I say, without it, and happily at that!

An Update

In the September 1977 A.R.E. Journal, my work in psoriasis appeared for the first time in a feature article entitled, *Psoriasis—Hope for the Afflicted*. In this account I reported on cases that had cleared and stayed clear for a three to four month period. An adequate amount of time had not yet elapsed before publication to observe whether or not there were to be any truly promising results as far as recurrence was concerned.

That was fourteen years ago. Surely, I would say, that is a reasonable amount of time to observe the validity of the treatment. The following is an update of these patients regarding their present state of health. Black and white photographs of their conditions appeared in Chapter 2, "Does It Work?"

1. In the Case of William (Bill) Culmone

Mr. Culmone, remember, was the first patient ever to follow the Cayce regimen under my care. After battling psoriasis for fifteen years, he followed the prescribed course as my first experiment and completely cleared in three months (from 7/25/75 to 10/16/75).

In a communication to me five months after we started treatments, Mrs. Culmone wrote the following:

> "Bill's psoriasis has cleared completely as a result of following the
> five points mentioned in conjunction with the office treatments
> (spinal adjustments). Bill was away ten days and did not take any
> medication with him. He followed his diet somewhat but did not
> have the sun, oil, colonic or herb treatments. We wanted to see if

the psoriasis would return. To date it has not returned. It is now just over five months since his first treatment. No signs of recurrence have been indicated. I, Minnie Culmone, wife of Bill, attest that we followed the treatments for psoriasis and the above statement is true."

After a period of one and one half years, Mr. Culmone was still clear. He remained clear until his unrelated death several years later.

2. *In the Case of Young A.S.*

He was virtually clear in a period of three to four months. Twelve years later, he has never really been bothered with the disease again. There have been some slight recurrences but nothing to speak of. His hands, chest and scalp remain clear even though he often strays from the diet.

3. *In the Case of Young E.L.*

She also cleared completely in a period of three to four months and has virtually remained clear after nine years. She is aware of eating the proper foods but, again, strays now and then but without any significant recurrence.

4. *In the Case of B.K.*

This was truly one of the most severe cases I have ever encountered. Practically every area of her body was severely afflicted. After suffering for two years, she cleared up in four months. Her thighs, elbows, scalp and especially her heels and bottoms of her feet, seemed to clear simultaneously. After ten years, she reported to me that she has never been troubled with the disease again. What slight flare up she might have, at times, is quickly resolved by going on the cleansing diet again. She has always been in control of her condition since she first cleared in 1977.

These are but a few of my early cases with a follow-up study several years after they were cleared. Little A.S. (now big A.S.!), along with baby E.L. (now beautiful teenager E.L.!), appear in my film, "Project: Psoriasis— Part I & II" which was produced in 1985, seven and eight years, respectively, after they cleared.

Their stories are heartwarming to say the least, offering true hope for those afflicted, especially in the case of children.

Teenagers—Take Heart!

One does not have to be a child psychologist to know it is no fun being a young person with psoriasis. Their greatest fear is feeling they will have to spend the rest of their lives going from one doctor to another, periodically being hospitalized in severe cases and never able to express their true personalities because of the inhibitions placed on them by the self-consciousness that accompanies psoriasis. Such a reaction is perfectly normal, for no one with a healthy mind wants to hide from life. Yet, they do hide to avoid embarrassment and thoughtless remarks from some of their peers.

A particular frustration is not being able to partake of teenage "junk" food with their friends. They may feel like an outcast which, in turn, leads to ever greater disappointment and undoubtedly produces internal toxins of its own accord. A vicious cycle is established. You're damned if you do and damned if you don't.

With some teenagers, however, depending on their attitude, there is no problem. True, they would like to enjoy the same foods and drinks as their friends, but they also understand and recognize the reason for their particular problem, so they stay away from such foods and avoid making it an issue. The strangest thing of all, however, is that after the first time or two in which they select only the foods that are permitted, *their friends don't care!* If they are harassed at first, an answer proven effective is to simply say, "I'd like to have that but, at the moment, I'm on a special Physical Fitness Diet." If the patient makes light of it, so will his or her friends. This produces a twofold benefit; they eat the proper foods while also realizing that they are just as well-liked by their friends for showing their individualism.

Do they still have to look upon the rest of their life with so many restrictions, particularly diet? Not necessarily. At the present time, I am coming closer to believing that, at least in some cases, the dietary restrictions can be lifted almost permanently if the patients stay on the regimen for at least six months after they clear. This fact has been mentioned in other chapters throughout this book, but the following account written by the mother of a teenager, B.M., who suffered a severe case of guttate psoriasis all over her body, should make teenagers take heart!

"My daughter B., started treatment with Dr. Pagano on January 7, 1983, after months of going to allergists and dermatologists. She was thirteen at the time and had psoriasis all over her body, on her head and on her face. The other doctors told me she would have to learn to live with it, and gave me creams to put on her skin which did not help. It is very hard for a thirteen year old to be told to live with such a disfigurement.

After six months treatment with Dr. Pagano, she cleared up, but then went off her diet and broke out again. She then resumed treatment and stayed on her diet. It has been two years since she cleared up with no recurrence. She also can eat anything she wants. Not a day goes by that I do not feel eternally grateful."

5/21/86   D.M.
(Date)   (Signed)

Having It Your Own Way

All psoriatics must keep in mind that they still may have a *tendency* toward the disease, even if every lesion on their body disappears by following this regimen. This should not be upsetting, and it usually isn't, for as stated earlier, the patients now have an understanding as to why it occurs and know what they must do to correct it. They can live free of the disease and live normal lives, provided they are willing to admit that their system reacts differently than others, particularly where certain foods are concerned. This is not unlike that of a diabetic or alcoholic; the difference being that psoriasis is far more controllable. They must learn to work with that fact rather than fight it, for, if they don't, they then will be fighting a losing battle. To insist on having an attitude of "I want what I want when I want it" is to seal their destiny to a lifetime of pain, disfigurement, mental anguish, and incredible expense. Instead, they should adopt the healthful attitude of "I will do all that is required of me"—and be thankful there is a way out of their dilemma. If they do, chances are in their favor that they will never again be concerned with the question of recurrence.

Chapter 21

Achieving The Goal
(A Mini-Review)

Before embarking on a regimen for the alleviation of any disease, I believe it advisable for the patient to understand not only the nature of the condition, but also the reasoning behind the course of therapy.

By way of review then, I advise my patients to always keep the following principles in mind:

1. Recognize psoriasis for what it is—the external manifestation of accumulated internal toxins.

2. The way to conquer the disease is by removing the toxins that have accumulated and prevent further contaminants from entering the system.

3. Toxins are removed and pollution is averted primarily by:
   a. Internal cleansing
   b. Proper dietary selection of food and drink

Other measures that help heal the intestinal walls such as: herb teas, spinal adjustments, oils, colonics, and the right mental attitude, etc., aid this process and will help one to achieve this goal of attaining clear skin in the shortest possible time.

The following is the basic procedure that I use for most of my patients. For others, as the need arises, I alter this regimen accordingly.

A. *The Apple Diet (The initial cleansing)*

Each day, for a period of three days, they eat nothing but Red Delicious or Golden Delicious apples (approximately 6 to 8) and drink 6 to 8 glasses of pure water. In addition, they take 1 to 2 ounces of pure olive oil each night followed by an enema.

On the third day, a colonic irrigation should be administered, if possible. Enemas may be given if colonics are unavailable.

This is the most effective way to begin the internal cleansing process. For details refer to Chapter 5, "Internal Cleansing."

B. *The Diet*

After having the colonic, they have a pint of plain yogurt. A few hours later, they eat a large green leafy salad. Dressing may be used but wine and grain vinegar is avoided. The dressing most preferred is olive oil combined with fresh lemon juice.

The dietary measures are continued as detailed in Chapter 6, "Diet and Nutrition." *Remember, Diet and proper Eliminations are the most important aspects of the regimen.* Six to eight glasses of pure water daily is essential.

C. *Epsom Salts Baths and Oils*

Hot Epsom Salts baths can be taken two or three times a week. However, this is not advised if one suffers from any kind of heart or circulatory condition or has skin with open sores that are cracked or sensitive.

An Epsom Salts bath is to be followed by an olive oil/peanut oil massage with the oils left on for at least 1/2 to 1 hour. The best results are achieved by leaving the oils on overnight. Wearing old, or inexpensive cotton garments over the oils has been found to be both comfortable and practical.

For thick, circumscribed lesions, castor oil, rubbed well into these areas, followed by an application of Cuticura or Hydrophilic Ointment has proved, in most cases, to be very effective. These products should be used daily until results are obtained. When improvement does occur, the patient cuts back on applying these substances to every other day. They discontinue use when the skin is cleared up. For more information, review my Chapter on "External Applications."

D. *The Herb Teas*

Slippery Elm Bark Powder and American Yellow Saffron Tea are the primary herb teas recommended. The alternatives are: Camomile, Mullein and Watermelon Seed Teas, which may be substituted period-ically for the Saffron Tea.

Slippery Elm Bark Powder is to be taken first thing in the morning. For severe cases, I have my patients drink it each morning for 10 days, then, every other morning for the next two weeks. Sometimes I have them refrain from taking it at all for the next full week. This cycle is repeated until the clearing takes place. In mild cases, it is taken every other day for three weeks and none on the fourth week. Again, the patient is to repeat this cycle until results are obtained. Slippery elm is not advised for pregnant women.

American Yellow Saffron Tea is to be taken in the afternoon and into the evening. A cup or two of freshly prepared saffron tea during this period is advised for mild cases. For severe cases, a teaspoon of saf-fron tea is prepared in a gallon of pure water, producing *saffron water*. It is used as the patient's drinking water whenever desired. As the lesions clear, it is no longer necessary to drink saffron water. However, the patient should still have a cup or two of saffron tea in the evening.

NOTE: If for any reason a patient cannot drink the Slippery Elm tea early in the morning, they may drink it at bedtime and have the Saffron Tea in the A.M. and though the day.

My chapter, "Herb Teas" details the preparation of these teas as I advise my patients.

E. *The Spinal Adjustments*

Spinal adjustments are usually administered after the first colonic and this process is to be continued once a week for twelve weeks. The treatments are centered on the *6th and 7th Dorsal*, *3rd Cervical*, *9th Dorsal*, and *4th Lumbar* vertebrae. They are to be adjusted only by a licensed chiropractor or osteopath. Stubborn cases will require a continuation of treatments until results are obtained.

For full details refer to Chapter, "The Role of the Spine."

F. *The Thought Process*

The correct psychology in getting well must always be the underlying common denominator for healing, especially when the patient is largely in control of his or her own regimen. Correct thinking and guarding one's thoughts from negative outside influences plays a vital role toward the road to recovery. Make no mistake about it; mental toxins in the form of anxiety, fear, resentment, etc., can turn the body acidic just as surely as does acid-forming foods—even more so.

Chapters "Right Thinking" and "The Emotional Factor" reinforces this concept.

REMEMBERING
The PURPOSE Behind
Each of the Six Basic SUGGESTIONS

SUGGESTION	*PURPOSE*
1. *Internal Cleansing:* Enemas, High Colonics, Fume, Steam and Epsom Salts baths, Cathartics (Laxatives), Plenty of Fresh Water.	To remove accumulated toxins (poisons) by improved bowel evacuation, adequate urinary drainage, and through the pores of the skin itself.
2. *The Proper Diet:* High alkaline (80%) to Less acid (20%). High-fiber, Fresh Fruit and Vegetables in particular.	Tends to keep the body chemistry more alkaline than acid. Helps improve evacuation as well as body building.
3. *Herb Teas:* Primarily, Slippery Elm Bark Powder and American Yellow Saffron Tea. Substitutes	Slippery Elm aids in the healing and rebuilding of the thin intestinal walls and helps prevent absorption of

for Saffron Tea: Camomile, Mullein and Watermelon Seed Tea.

toxins. Saffron helps repair of intestinal walls, acts as an intestinal antiseptic, flushes out the liver and kidneys and removes toxins through the perspiratory (sweat) glands if taken prior to a steam bath.

4. *Spinal Adjustments:* Centered on (in order of importance): 6th & 7th Dorsal, 3rd Cervical, 9th Dorsal, and 4th Lumbar vertebrae.

Insures proper nerve impulses and circulation to the walls of the upper intestinal tract as well as the glandular centers.

5. *External Applications:* Oils, Ointments, Baths, Steam, Massage.

Helps soothe the external lesions, keeping them soft and pliable. Helps reduce scaling, relieve itching and heal the surface cells.

6. *Right Thinking:*

Helps keep the mind focused on the healing process rather than on the disease.

Each patient is advised to "see", in their mind's eye, the purpose for each suggestion actually taking place as they are carried out. This aids the healing process by practicing the Art of VISUALIZATION.

Patience and *Persistence* is the key to all the aforementioned procedures. Without these qualities, one cannot even hope to achieve a satisfactory result, especially one that is lasting. It is important to keep in mind just how long one has struggled and lived with this disease and how much psoriasis has dominated his or her life. The patients who have been successful by following the prescribed regimen feel that the time and sacrifice that they have made, in order to rid themselves of this disease, is but a small price to pay to have this burden lifted from their shoulders.

Chapter 22

QUO VADIS?
(Where Do We Go From Here?)

Needed: The Ideal Psoriasis Center

The photographic results depicted in this book have more significance than meets the eye. Of course, first and foremost, they prove the theory works—for many people—but just as profound is the fact that these results were obtained under the *worst* conditions. By that I mean, there was no direct daily control. The patients were told what to do and were expected to go home and do it. Except for the spinal adjustments once a week that could only take place in the office, the patients were largely on their own.

On each visit their progress was noted, concepts reinforced, and whenever possible, personal meetings with other patients who were successful were arranged. I mark this fact as significant in that if results such as those depicted herein were possible without complete control, how much more successful would they be under hospital or clinical auspices? All the measures would be able to be administered with the proper equipment, ingredients and attitudes. Ideally, such a center should be located near the sea where there is plenty of fresh air and sunshine and as pollution-free as possible.

Patients would come to such a center to *learn*, as well as to have the therapies administered over a two to four week period. After the patient's initial stay, they would then have the knowledge of how to handle their problem and return home to continue to carry out the procedures.

A two to four week stay might show a significant change in the skin, *but not necessarily so*. The chances are the change will not be as dramatic as PUVA or the Goeckerman treatment. They have been shown to apparently clear the skin almost completely in that period of time—and, in some cases, they may remain clear for many months. In just as many cases, however, the condition returned shortly afterward and in full force, worse than before. Desperation is the understandable aftereffect, not to mention the fact that with such therapy, the patient is always dependent on hospital control.

The idea of a psoriasis center of this nature, I feel, would be much in demand and highly valuable to the psoriatic. "Patience and Persistence" in *all* matters, may one day make such a center a reality.

The Future—A Choice

Let's say the patients have followed the regimen and are successful. The lesions have completely disappeared. Their skin is beautiful. They feel confident and proud of themselves. What now? Will psoriasis return? Are they really cured of the malady or will it hang over their heads forever?

The answer to these questions depend a great deal on how one interprets the word "cure." Blakiston's New Gould Medical Dictionary describes "cure" as "to heal or make well." It is the successful treatment of an illness or wound.

To be "cured" of a disease does not mean it could never return particularly if the patient resumes the lifestyle or conditions that brought it about in the first place. It means the malady has been corrected—that, obviously, the course of therapy employed was effective in bringing about a cure or healing.

In cases of psoriasis, the patient does have a choice. This is not necessarily true for all diseases. He may choose to ignore the basic rules of proper hygiene and sound reasoning pertaining to his former illness and bring about a resurgence of the problem, or he could react with gratitude, respect his body, appreciate it and learn to prevent further episodes of ill-health for the remainder of his life. This, to me, is the person who is "cured." The healing was physically, mentally and spiritually complete.

Once the patient's skin is clear, most cases that I have treated successfully later fall into one or a combination of the following categories:

Group I

They will be eternally grateful and remain on the regimen practically as a way of life and, more than likely, always remain clear.

Group II

They will remain faithful to the basic regimen "for the most part"— but periodically eat whatever they enjoy.

This attitude prevails with the majority of patients and I am not necessarily against it. Let's face it—we want to enjoy our lives; food and drink is part of that enjoyment. With some, however, living to eat far overshadows eating to live. Satisfying one's desire for certain viands may prevent frustration from setting in, which in itself is a leading cause of toxic buildup with emotional origins. With this group, however, panic no longer exists. They *know* what works to rid themselves of lesions the minute they begin to "pop out."

Group III

They realize it can be completely alleviated so they go back to their old ways of eating and drinking. In time, the lesions will return, usually worse than before; as with Group II, they won't panic. Having been successful once, they feel they can take over and be in control whenever they decide to get around to it. The sad part about this group is—they never do! Those patients find no sympathy with me. They seem to forget that there is a law of irreversibility. One day the organs of the emunctory system will, because of overtaxation, break down to the point of no return.

This group should hear as often as I do, the plea of those they live with who suffer the silent burden of "clean up" wherever the psoriatic goes.

How often I have heard, "Doctor, everyday, all day, in order to keep my home presentable, I have to follow my husband around with a vacuum cleaner. In the morning, I scoop up scales in our bed as I would scoop up snow or sand on the beach. It is driving me crazy."

True, the psoriasis patient has a problem, but so do those they live with. To some devoted and sincere people, their complaining about their loved one's condition may seem selfish and therefore, refrain from voicing their true feelings. This is nothing compared to the selfishness on the part of the patient who chooses not to control his or her problem when there is a strong possibility that they can.

To these unfortunate psoriatics, I say, turn the tide by making those around them the center of *their* concern. Who knows? Such a thoughtful act may, in itself, lead to a miracle. In other words, it is the patient who is doing something for somebody else.

Group IV

They will combine the efforts of Medicine and Cayce which could bring about incredible results. As soon as possible, however, they should lean more toward the natural alternative and avoid orthodox procedures that may have serious side effects.

Group V

They usually revert back to orthodox management if their nature is to be totally undisciplined, which, in extreme cases, can mean a series of hospital stays for the rest of their lives.

The patient, you see, has to *decide* what is the most important factor in his life. Does he really want to get rid of the disease or doesn't he? Is the effort to change his lifestyle really worth it? This must be determined for the decision will strongly influence the final outcome.

In all fairness, it has been my experience to observe that the vast majority of patients do truly wish to be healed. This attitude makes all the years of study, effort, experimentation and risk, worth the price. If successful, the patient is always delighted, but as a physician, I can think of no greater reward than that glow of happiness, that sense of accomplishment, that comes with the knowledge that....

My Patient Is Well!

Testimonials & Professional Endorsements

From the Patients:

"I have been treated for psoriasis by a supposed prominent physician in Manhattan. The treatment was costly and ineffective. Dr. Pagano's procedure works for me and is a great therapy that I firmly believe should work for everyone."

> Mr. T. S. M.
> New York City

"For over 10 years I had been searching for a medical miracle, only to find temporary relief from psoriasis. Thanks to Dr. Pagano's years of research, I no longer suffer from this skin disease. There is only *one* cure and that is a natural one through nutrition."

> Miss D. M.
> New York City

"I went to so many doctors for 25 years and got tired of needles and medicines; they never did any good. I only got worse. Dr. Pagano's method is natural. I'm not putting any drugs in my system. I'm comfortable with it. Now, after following his therapy, the psoriasis I was plagued with is practically gone."

> Miss M. V.
> Little Ferry, NJ

"Thanks to Dr. Pagano's healing system, the skin on my hands is virtually free of psoriasis after 20 years of discomfort and limited activity. Conventional therapies never worked."

Mr. J. W. E.
Woodstock, NY

"When I first went to see Dr. Pagano I had a terrible case of psoriasis. I had already been to several skin doctors in the state of New Jersey. After reviewing my case, Dr. Pagano put me on a diet of natural foods, herb teas, chiropractic adjustments and internal cleansing. I never felt better in my life. After about three months it all started to clear up. That was thirteen years ago. I find it pays to stick to the diet. I am very happy with the results."

Mrs. P. G.
Hilton Head Island, SC

"Psoriasis began on the back of my right leg. It continually spread until it engulfed my entire right ankle. My medical doctor diagnosed it as psoriasis and recommended I see Dr. Pagano. Through diet and chiropractic adjustments I found relief from the itching and gradual healing of this skin disease. I often met and spoke with other patients of his that had similar successes."

Mrs. N. O.
Scotch Plains, NJ

From the Professionals:

"Many years ago, the mystic, Edgar Cayce, came up with an effective, holistic treatment for psoriasis, an incurable skin disease. Dr. John Pagano, in this illustrated volume, shows us how he has been helping psoriasis sufferers in a natural way—the Edgar Cayce way. Victims of this disease and others may well marvel at the results."

JESS STEARN
Author of the Best Seller,
Edgar Cayce—The Sleeping Prophet
Malibu, CA

"Edgar Cayce, and the research conducted by Dr. Pagano, unveils the mystery of psoriasis, one of mankind's oldest skin diseases. This book opens the door for further research, bringing forth undeniable evidence that psoriasis may no longer be considered 'incurable'."

JOHN G. FULLER
Author/Journalist
Weston, CONN.

"Dr. John Pagano, in this book on psoriasis, has articulated the essence of Cayce's philosophy and theories of illness and applied them faithfully to one of society's most emotionally and socially debilitating afflictions with amazing results. This work will have profound influence on how we will view the healing process in the future."

JAMES C. WINDSOR, Ed.D., LL.D.
Past Pres., Edgar Cayce Foundation
Williamsburg, VA

"I have viewed the evidence, I have met Dr. Pagano's patients—it works! This book should encourage further research not only in psoriasis and the dermatoses, but in other devastating illnesses. Responsible researchers would do well to seriously investigate this material for what it has to offer suffering humanity."

FAINA MUNITS, M.D., Ph.D.
West Orange, NJ

APPENDIXES

APPENDIX A—Nutritional Considerations

    a.   80% / 20% Food Ratio

    b.   Avoid List

    c.   Above Ground/Below Ground Food Chart

    d.   Proteins and Starches

    e.   Principles on Breakfast, Lunch and Dinner

    f.   Sample Daily Menu

    g.   Food Combinations to Avoid

    h.   Reminders

APPENDIX B—Self-Hypnosis Recording for the Psoriatic

APPENDIX C—Product Suppliers

NUTRITIONAL
CONSIDERATIONS
IN THE
NATURAL HEALING
OF
PSORIASIS, ECZEMA AND PSORIATIC ARTHRITIS

Approval by your personal
physician is essential
before embarking on any
dietary program.

Avoid any food item
that causes an allergic
reaction even if it is
on the permitted list.

80% of the Daily Food Intake Should be Selected From the Following:

WATER:

- 6 to 8 glasses of pure water daily

FRUIT:

Fresh preferred, Frozen is permitted, Packed in water in glass jars, on occasion.

- Allowed: Apples (cooked), Apricots, Most Berries, Cherries, Dates, Figs (unsulphured), Grapes, Grapefruit, Lemons, Limes, Mango, Nectarines, Oranges, Papaya, Peaches, Pears, Pineapple, Prunes (small), etc.

NOTE: Raw Apples, Bananas & Melons are permitted provided they are eaten alone and sparingly.

- Permitted in lesser quantities are: Avocado, Cranberries, Currants, Large Prunes & Plums.

VEGETABLES:

Fresh preferred, Frozen are permitted, Packed in glass jars on occasion. (Daily Intake should be 3 that grow above the ground to 1 that grows below the ground.)

- Allowed: Asparagus, Beets, Broccoli, Brussel Sprouts, Carrots*, Celery*, Cucumbers, Garlic*, Lettuce* (Romaine in particular), Onions*, Parsnips, Scallions, Soy Beans, Spinach*, Sprouts*, String Beans, Squash, Sweet Potatoes, Watercress*.

NOTE: Those marked with (*) are particularly important.

- Permitted in lesser quantities are: White Corn, Dried Beans, Peas, Lentils & Rhubarb.

20% *of the Daily Food Intake Should be Selected From the Following*:

GRAINS:

- All grains should be whole grain, natural products such as: Breads, Bagels, Muffins, Cereals with very little, if any, preservatives or artificial sweeteners. (No White Flour Products.)

MEATS:

- *Chicken & Turkey* (skinless, white meat preferred)

- *Fish* (not shellfish)—Cold, salt water, white flesh varieties preferred. Fresh or frozen.

- *Lamb*—Trimmed of all fat before cooking, well done, about twice a week.

  NOTE: The above listed meats are never to be fried. No more than 4 to 6 oz. is permitted at a serving—once a day. Poultry may be cooked with the skin intact but then the skin is to be removed before eating.

DAIRY:

- Only *Lowfat/ Low Sodium* products are permitted: Skim or Lowfat Milk, Cheese, Buttermilk, Yogurt, etc. (No Ice Cream, Cream Toppings or Whole Milk Products.)

  NOTE: In cases of Eczema, Goat's Milk and Soy Milk are suggested.

- *Butter* (regular) is permitted but only occasionally and in very sparing amounts. *Eggs* are permitted, 2 to 4 per week, prepared any way but fried.

- All products high in saturated fat are to be avoided.

- Do not have Citrus Fruits or Citrus Juices with Dairy products or Cereals at the same meal.

It is important to adhere to the 80%/20% food selection in order to maintain a proper Acid/Base Balance, but avoid any food item that causes an allergic reaction.

AVOID AVOID AVOID

- *All Red Meats* (except Lamb): Beef, Pork, Veal, Sweetbreads, etc.

- *Processed Meats*: Sausage, Salami, Bologna, etc.

- *The Nightshades*: Tomatoes (and Tomato sauces), Tobacco (smoking), Eggplant, Peppers, White Potatoes, Paprika

- *Shellfish*: Lobster, Shrimp, Clams, Crabs, etc., and sauces made with shellfish.

- *Alcoholic beverages*

- All Fried Foods, Pizza, Soda (diet & regular), Sweets and Pastries, Sugary Cereals, Chocolate, Gravies, Wine or Grain (white) Vinegar and Hot Spices.

- "Junk" Food and Fast Food Items such as, Candy, Potato Chips, French Fries, Hamburgers, Hot Dogs, Vending Machine Foods, Foods made with a great deal of artificial flavorings, colorings and preservatives, etc.

ABOVE/BELOW GROUND VEGETABLES

Most vegetables, as well as fruits, are alkaline formers and purifiers of the blood. Vegetables should be chosen and consumed on a daily basis in proportion to 3 that grow above the ground to 1 that grows below the ground. Examples of above and below ground vegetables follow (vegetables that are prohibited are not listed):

ABOVE GROUND (3)

ARTICHOKE • ASPARAGUS • BEANS (SOY, LENTILS, PEAS) • BROCCOLI • BRUSSEL SPROUTS • CABBAGE • CAULIFLOWER • CELERY • CHICORY • CHIVES • CUCUMBER • DANDELION • ENDIVE • FENNEL • LEEKS • LETTUCE (ALL TYPES) • OLIVE • PARSLEY • PUMPKIN • SPINACH • WATERCRESS • ZUCCHINI

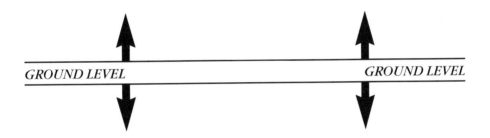

GROUND LEVEL   *GROUND LEVEL*

BELOW GROUND (1)

BEETS • CARROTS • GARLIC • JERUSALEM ARTICHOKE (SUNCHOKE) • ONIONS • OYSTER PLANT (SALSIFY, GOATSBEARD) • RADISHES • SWEET POTATOES • TURNIPS

<u>NOTE</u>: *Onions, as well as Lettuce, Celery, Spinach and Carrots are particularly recommended.*

PROTEINS AND STARCHES

Below are listed proteins and starches that are permitted in the diet, but should not be combined to too great an extent with each other at the same meal.

Proteins	*Starches*
Fish, Fowl and Lamb	All Cereals
Cheese	Dry Beans and Peas
Eggs	Breads and Crackers
Milk	Bran
All Types of Grains	Corn and Rice
Nuts	Syrups and Sugars (use only those permitted)
Dried Beans, Peas, Soybeans & Lentils	Squash (winter), Pumpkin & Yams
Avocado	Grains: Barley, Buckwheat, Millet, Oats, Rye, etc.
Olives	Beets, Burdock, Carrots, Parsnips, Rutabaga, Salsify (Oyster Plant), Water Chestnuts—(All Alkaline-Reacting)

Note: Some items are listed in both columns because they are a protien as well as a starch.

PRINCIPLES ON BREAKFAST, LUNCH AND DINNER

SUGGESTED BREAKFAST MEALS

The Slippery Elm drink should be taken at least 1/2 hour before breakfast for best results, unless it was taken the night before.

Most breakfast foods in the American diet are to a large extent acid-formers, therefore, should not be consumed in very large portions. Foods such as whole-grain cereals (hot or cold), breads, muffins, pancakes, etc. are acid-forming, whereas, other desirable breakfast foods such as, stewed fruits, baked apple, stewed figs, stewed raisins, and stewed apricots are alkaline-forming.

Hot cereals should not be cooked too long, as this would destroy the vitamins and minerals necessary for building greater resistance in the body. Any non-citrus fruit, chopped or slivered almonds, or a little honey or pure maple syrup may be added to hot or cold cereal.

Citrus fruits and citrus fruit juices (primarily orange and grapefruit) remember, must not be eaten at the same meal with cereals, gruels or dairy products. Citrus may be eaten alone unless the patient experiences a reaction, such as itching, rash, or hypersensitivity of any kind. If this occurs, I advise my patients to curtail or eliminate citrus from their diet altogether, at least for the time being.

The most desirable fruit juices are those of the non-citrus variety, such as, apricot, pear, grape, apple, mango, papaya and the like. Cranberry is acid-forming.

Keep in mind that raw apples, bananas, and melons, although permitted on the diet, should be eaten alone, that is, by themselves, as a snack between meals, but not eaten at the same meal with other foods.

Eggs (two to four per week) are permitted, unless the patient is on a special low cholesterol diet. Even at that, they may only be prepared by boiling (preferably soft-boiled or coddled), steamed, or cooked in a teflon pan without oil or fat of any kind.

Milk, cheese, yogurt, buttermilk, etc. should always be of the lowfat or nonfat and low salt variety. Skim milk and skim milk products are preferred.

Coffee is permitted, but it should be "black", that is, without cream or sugar, naturally decaffeinated, and no more than three cups per day. Some patients have substituted a cup of hot water with the juice of a fresh lemon in the morning in place of coffee.

Jelly preserves, 100% pure, without preservatives or additives, may be spread lightly on whole-grain toast or English Muffins in place of butter or margarine.

These "rules" may seem new to many patients, but soon they get the idea and before long it becomes second nature to them and they proceed without difficulty.

SUGGESTED LUNCHEON MEALS

Lunch should consist primarily of fresh, raw, green leafy vegetables, especially Celery, Spinach, Watercress, and all types of Lettuce, particularly Romaine, at least four times a week. Olive oil and fresh lemon juice is the preferred salad dressing. Ingredients such as, a little water-packed, White-Meat Tuna, Sliced White Meat Turkey or Chicken Breast, Hard-Boiled Eggs, Tofu, Feta, Lowfat Cottage Cheese, and other types of Salt-Free Lowfat Cheese may be added on occasion for variety. A good alternate is a fresh fruit salad. If desired, a cup of home-made fat free soup or broth may be included as part of the luncheon meal.

Freshly grated or finely chopped vegetables such as, Carrots, Celery, Beets, Watercress, etc. *combined in gelatin* and served on a bed of green, leafy vegetables is also highly suggested, as are fresh fruits and their juices in gelatin. The nutrients contained in these foods, when combined in gelatin, are absorbed and assimilated by the body to a much greater degree. These particular types of salads may also be chosen as a luncheon meal or eaten as a snack at any time.

SUGGESTED DINNER MEALS

Dinner should consist of a raw vegetable salad, at least two or three cooked vegetables, and no more than a 6 oz. portion of Fish, Lamb or Poultry. By cooking vegetables in Patapar or Vegetable Parchment Paper, they are baked in their own juices, thereby retaining all their vital nutrients. This method of cooking vegetables is preferred above all others, however, they may also be Steamed, Baked, Microwaved, Pressure-Cooked or Stir-Fried. It should be noted that Stir-Frying does not mean frying foods in large amounts of oils or fats, but is rather the Oriental method of quickly cooking diced, chopped or shredded foods, such as meats, fish, chicken, turkey or vegetables in a Wok or heavy skillet for a few minutes, or until tender, in very little oil. Shortening, Refined Fats and Oils (Unsaturated as well as Saturated) should never be used when cooking foods. It is best not to over-cook vegetables or deep-fry them.

Remember—each meal is important. They should not be skipped.

SAMPLE DAILY MENU

PURE WATER—6 to 8 Glasses Daily

LECITHIN—1 Tablespoon, three times a day until condition clears, then reduce to 1 Tablespoon per day. Do not take Lecithin more than 5 days per week. Granular Lecithin may be added to foods and liquids.

BREAKFAST

- *1/2 HOUR BEFORE BREAKFAST*: 1 Cup of Slippery Elm Bark Powder Tea—OR—1 Slippery Elm Lozenge. [For Preparation of Teas—Refer to Chapter "HERB TEAS."]

- 1 Glass of Pure Water

- Grape, Pear, Apricot, Papaya or any other Non-Citrus Fruit Juice [4 oz.].

- 1 Bowl of Dry or Cooked Whole-Grain Cereal [Skim Milk, Natural Sweeteners and/or any Non-Citrus—Alkaline-Forming Fruit may be added except Apples, Bananas, Melons, and Dried or Stewed Fruits].

- 1 Whole-Grain Muffin, Bagel or Slice of Bread, Toasted. [A pat of Unsalted Butter or Cold-Pressed Margarine may be added and, if desired, 1 Teaspoon of Natural Fruit Jelly or Honey.]

- 1 Cup of Black-Decaffeinated Coffee—1 Cup of Hot Water with Lemon Juice—1 Glass of Skim Milk [Select 1].

MID-MORNING SNACK, If Desired: [Select 1 or 2]

Apple—Banana—Fruit Juice—Plain Lowfat Yogurt—Dried Unsulphured Fruit—A Few Almonds

LUNCH

- 1 Glass of Pure Water

- Raw Fresh Vegetable Salad with Olive Oil/Lemon Juice Dressing, Seasoned with Fresh Herbs [If desired—Small portions of either

Skinless, White Meat Chicken, Turkey, Water-Packed Tuna or Lowfat Cheese may be added]

- Plain Lowfat Yogurt—OR—1 Whole-Grain Cookie—OPTIONAL

- 1 Cup of Black-Decaffeinated Coffee—1 Cup of Hot Water with Fresh Lemon or Lime Juice—1 Glass of Skim Milk—1 Glass of Seltzer, Perrier or Saratoga Water with a wedge of Lemon or Lime [Select 1]

[OR]

- 1 Glass of Pure Water

- 1 Cup of Salt-Free Bouillon—OR—1 Cup of Home-Made Vegetable Soup [Lightly Seasoned and without Tomato]—OPTIONAL

- Fresh Fruit Salad on a Bed of Lettuce and a small portion of Lowfat Cottage Cheese [May be served plain or with Lowfat Yogurt Dressing]

MID-AFTERNOON SNACK, If Desired: [Select 1 or 2]

Whole-Grain Rice Cake [Plain or with 1 Teaspoon of Honey or Natural Fruit Jelly]—Fruit Juice—1 Slice of Melon—1 Cup of Fat-Free and Salt-Free Broth—100% Natural Frozen Fruit Bar—1 Cup of American Yellow Saffron Tea

DINNER

- *1/2 HOUR BEFORE DINNER*: 1 Glass of 100% Pure Grape Juice—OPTIONAL

- 1 Glass of Pure Water

- 1 Cup of Home-made Barley Soup—OR—1 Cup of Brown Rice Soup [Lightly Seasoned, Fat-Free and Preferably, Salt-Free]—OPTIONAL

- Cooked (Preferably, Steamed) Vegetables [Include a variety of Above and Below Ground, Yellow and Green Vegetables]

- Small Fresh Green Vegetable Salad (Mixed Greens) with a sprinkling of Olive Oil and Lemon Juice—OPTIONAL

- Fish, Poultry (Skinless) or Lamb—4 to 6 oz., Trimmed of all Fat [Poached, Broiled, Steamed or Baked—DO NOT FRY]

- Baked Apple (sweetened with 1 Teaspoon of Honey or Pure Maple Syrup, if desired)—Fresh Fruit—Natural Fruit Ice [Select 1]

- 1 Cup of Herb Tea (Camomile, Mullein or Watermelon Seed)—1 Cup of Black-Decaffeinated Coffee (No Sugar)—1 Cup of Hot Water with Fresh Lemon or Lime Juice—1 Glass of Seltzer, Perrier, or Saratoga Water with a wedge of Lemon or Lime [Select 1]

EVENING SNACK, If Desired: [Select 1 or 2]

1 Glass of Fruit Juice—1 Whole-Grain Cookie—1 Fresh Fruit (Peach, Tangerine, Orange, Nectarine, etc.)—1 Cup of Stewed Fruit

BEFORE BEDTIME: 1 Cup of American Yellow Saffron Tea

NOTE: Slippery Elm Tea and Saffron Tea may be reversed by drinking Saffron Tea 1/2 hour before breakfast and Slippery Elm Tea before bedtime.

FOOD COMBINATIONS TO AVOID

Most people are not aware that certain foods should not be combined at the same meal, but may, if desired, be eaten separately. This is because some food combinations may cause havoc within the body that sooner or later show their deleterious effect in the form of poor digestion as well as improper utilization and assimilation of vital nutrients. When this occurs, the end result is intestinal discomfort, malnutrition and poor elimination. Add the over-abundance of acid-formers and you have the breeding ground for a generalized toxic build-up. The following food combinations are therefore to be avoided for the very reasons just stated. When preparing meals, the proper 80% alkaline—20% acid ratio should always be kept in mind.

- Do not combine whole-grain products, i.e. cereals, breads, etc. with citrus fruits, citrus juices, or stewed and dried fruits.

- Do not combine citrus fruits or their juices with dairy products, such as cheese, milk or yogurt.

- Do not combine any type of fruit with white flour products, such as bread, crackers, cereals, pasta, etc.

- Do not combine melons (any variety), raw apples or bananas with other foods. These fruits may, however, be eaten separately.

- Do not add milk, cream or sugar to coffee or tea.

- Do not combine too many Acid-Forming foods (Proteins, Starches, Sugars, Fats and Oils) at the same meal.

REMINDERS

- The suggested amount of water intake, 6 to 8 glasses of pure water daily, is *in addition* to all other beverages, i.e. juice, tea, coffee, etc.

- Granular Lecithin may be added to beverages or sprinkled on foods.

- The Herb Teas are best consumed without adding milk, cream or sugar. A teaspoon of lemon juice or a teaspoon of honey may be added if desired.

- It is best to drink American Yellow Saffron Tea more often than the other suggested herbal teas. This tea should not be consumed, however, too soon after taking Slippery Elm Tea. A time lapse of several hours between drinking these particular teas is suggested.

- Milk, cream or sugar should not be added to Naturally Decaffeinated Coffee. No more than 3 cups per day is permitted.

- The primary cleansers of the body are fruit and fruit juices, pure water, and the herbal teas; whereas, the primary builders of the body are vegetables and vegetable juices. These "cleansers and builders" are the mainstay of the diet. The relatively few fruits and vegetables that are acid-forming need not be of too much concern unless a decided adverse reaction occurs. If so, they should be avoided. Learn how to listen to your own body.

- In-between meal snacks are optional.

- Always choose foods carefully when preparing a daily or weekly menu. Try to vary your selection of foods in order to prevent a feeling of deprivation or boredom.

- It is best to use sparing amounts of spices, sweeteners, butter, margarine and oils when cooking or adding to foods.

- Acidic and blood cholesterol levels are reduced by limiting fat and sugar intake.

- Foods that cause an allergic reaction should be avoided even if they appear on the "Permitted" food list.

- Carbonated drinks, especially regular and diet soda, are not permitted. The only exception is Seltzer (not Club Soda) or Naturally-Carbonated Spring Waters to which may be added lemon or lime juice. Even these beverages should be consumed only on an occasional basis.

- Fresh fruits, vegetables and high-fiber foods are the best sources of maintaining adequate, daily bowel eliminations. In addition to these foods, home enemas or natural cathartics often aid in cases of chronic constipation. High colonic irrigations should be professionally administered and only with the approval of a licensed physician.

- Red or white wine, 2—4 oz., may be consumed once in awhile, but only if one is not on any type of medication or suffers from Gout.

- All dairy products such as, milk, cheese, yogurt, etc. should be skim or lowfat varieties and consumed only in moderate amounts.

- A good substitute for a cup of coffee is a cup of hot water with the juice of a lemon or lime.

- Over-eating is never advocated even with the foods that are allowed. Eat less—live longer!

APPENDIX B

SELF-HYPNOSIS RECORDING for the PSORIATIC

The following discourse is the basis for a self-hypnosis cassette tape that I and a professional hypnotist developed for a certain few of my psoriasis patients. With specific alterations, depending on the patient, it can be adapted to meet the needs of each individual.

Most important is that the patient record the entire message *in their own voice*, twice on the same tape with about a ten second pause in between. This allowed the message to enter their mind just before sleep set in and permitted the patient to turn off the tape player without having to rewind. In the morning, upon awakening, they simply place the ear phones back on and press the "play" button and the same message is repeated. In this way the patient receives the message at those periods when the subconscious mind is most amenable to suggestions.

I repeat, this segment of the regimen *is not for everyone*. It is placed here only to give my readers and professionals an idea of the basic principles involved. Most of my patients do not need this added technique. They carry out the measures without implementing the aid of a self-hypnosis tape.

Psoriasis Self-Hypnosis Tape:

"I close my eyes...(pause), then I take three deep breaths...(pause for three deep breaths). I will count backward from 10 to 1, feeling more and more relaxed with every number and every breath I take.

(count) "10—9—8—7—6—5—4—3—2—1

"Following my special cleansing diet is the easiest thing in the world for me to do. I desire to eat only the foods that I know are good for me. I look upon most animal fats, sweets, hard alcohol and the nightshades, especially tomatoes, as unhealthy to my body, therefore, I have no problem in avoiding them. It does not bother me in the least that other people can tolerate them. I know they are simply not for me. I do enjoy, however, chicken, fish and lamb prepared any way except fried. I avoid fried foods completely.

"When thirsty, I am quickly satisfied with a glass of pure water or seltzer with the juice of a fresh lime or lemon, with or without ice, knowing it is very tasty and cleansing.

(For heavy smokers): "I am gradually cutting down the number of cigarettes I smoke for I recognize tobacco as a nightshade, therefore should be avoided. I am quite satisfied with just 3 or 4 cigarettes a day and see myself eliminating them altogether very soon. I find that I can feel satisfied by substituting a drink of water or seltzer for a cigarette.

"I am enjoying my life more and more knowing each passing day I am cleaning out unnecessary poisons and acids that my body does not need, with improved bowel and bladder evacuation.

"I know that green, leafy vegetables and fresh fruits are not only highly nutritious, but aid greatly in the evacuation of the bowel and kidneys and I enjoy eating them regularly. They help bring the body into a normal balance, filling me with more energy. As my skin clears, I focus my attention on the areas that have cleared or are clearing. If it clears in one part of my body, I know it can clear in *all* parts of my body. I joyfully allow my body all the time it needs and visualize myself totally clear.

"I have grown above stressful conditions by learning how to 'take things lightly.' This does not mean I minimize important matters. It means I give everything the attention it deserves, and no more. I know I can handle any situation that comes into my life, thereby making the best possible use of my energy. I am content to do what I can, then leave the rest to take care of itself. This is not only accomplishing my goals, but doing it in an enjoyable, relaxed way.

"Each new day is now an adventure for me, one in which I allow only constructive, healthy thoughts to enter my consciousness. As I reflect on my former life-style, I recognize the changes as they occur in my life in the form of revitalized health, renewed ambition and restored energy.

"Every time I hear this recorded message it is deeply engraved into my subconscious and consequently manifests in my everyday life.

"I will now count forward from 1 to 10. At the count of 10 I will open my eyes, feeling well-rested, and turn off the recorder. I have renewed motivation to achieve my goal of freeing myself of psoriasis every time I listen to this personal message.

"1—2—3—4—5—6—7—8—9—10

Turn off the recorder."

(Author's note: Henry Leo Bolduc, author of the book, *Self-Hypnosis: Creating Your Own Destiny*, has now made available, through the A.R.E., a course on cassette tape, *How to Get Results Through Self-Hypnosis*— Details may be obtained by writing to the A.R.E. Bookstore, Virginia Beach, Virginia 23451.)

APPENDIX C

PRODUCT SUPPLIERS

The following suppliers have available the most important items required for Psoriasis, Psoriatic Arthritis and Eczema. They include: Slippery Elm Bark Powder—American Yellow Saffron Tea—Glyco-Thymoline—Atomodine—The Tri Salts (Sulfur, Cream of Tartar, Rochelle Salts) Trade names, "Purilax" at Home Health Products; "Sulflax" at Heritage Store,—also—Almond Glow or Aura Glow (both Olive Oil/Peanut Oil Mixtures) and Castor Oil.

Home Health Products, Inc.   -or-
(Official supplier)
(1160 A Millers Lane)
P.O. Box 3130
Virginia Beach, VA 23454

Tel: (804) 491-2200
Mail order: (800) 284-9123

The Heritage Store
(314 Laskin Road)
P.O. Box 444
Virginia Beach, VA 23458

Tel: (804) 428-0100
Mail Order: (800) 862-2923

(Catalogs available on request)

Most other items; such as, Cuticura Products, Hydrophilic Ointment, Epsom Salts, Witch Hazel, etc. are obtained or ordered from local pharmacies.

SUBJECT MATTER BY CHAPTER

CHAPTER 5
Internal Cleansing

Starting from the beginning—Opening the normal channels of elimination—Chronic constipation and poor eliminative habits—Francis M. Pottenger, M.D.—The Colon (Large Intestine)—Fig. 5-1—Abnormal Shapes of the Bowel—Fig. 5-2A, Fig. 5-2B, Fig. 5-2C—Bernard Jensen, D.C., Ph.D.—Bad Toilet Habits—Different diseases, same cause?—Begin with Internal Cleansing—The Kidneys—The Position of the Kidneys—Fig. 5-3—Dialysis—The Skin and Lungs—The Skin—The Lungs—The Position of the Lungs—Fig. 5-4—The Liver—The Position of the Liver—Fig. 5-5—The Liver/Skin-Kidney/Lung Correlation—Henry G. Bieler, M.D.—Effective Cleansing Measures—The High Colonic Irrigation—Home Enemas—A Patient's Technique for a Home Enema—Preliminary Diet to the Colonic or Home Enema—The Three Day Apple Diet (modified)—Apples—Not for Everyone—Alternatives to the Apple Diet—The Grape Diet—The Citrus Diet—The Fresh Fruit Diet—The Importance of Water—Natural Cathartics (Laxatives)—Best and Taylor on Vitamin B—Effective Combinations—Fletcher's Castoria—Syrup of Figs—Orange Juice Sandwich—Other natural eliminants—Olive Oil—Glyco-Thymoline—The Tri-Salts (Sulphur, Cream of Tartar and Rochelle Salts)—High Fiber Foods—Detoxification—Fume and Steam Baths—Fig. 5-6, A Steam cabinet in use—Saffron and Steam—Exercise—Toxins—Pottenger—Improved Bathroom Facilities—Auto-intoxication—The "Glut" Response—Thoughts and Toxins 39

CHAPTER 6
Diet and Nutrition
(Basics)

The importance of diet as it pertains to psoriasis—Cayce's discourse # 2455-2—A renewed interest in nutrition—The Acid/Alkaline Balance—The 80%/20% Food Ratio—Alkaline Formers vs. Acid Formers—Alkaline Formers—Fruits accorded special attention—Vegetables—Beware, The Nightshades!—Measures that increase alkalinity—Acid Formers—Acid Forming Foods—Measures that increase acidity—The Effect Toxemia Has on the Acid/Alkaline (Base) Balance-Pottenger—Glyco-Thymoline—Lecithin—Lecithin and Psoriasis—Adelle Davis—Case in Point—Atmospheric Influence on the Acid/Alkaline Balance—Avoiding the Nightshades—Norman F. Childers, Ph.D., The Nightshades—Pizza—Salad Dressings—Olive Oil—Shellfish—Fish—Poultry (Fowl)—Lamb—Dairy Products—Grains—Sweets—For the Sweet Tooth—Carob—Artificial Sweeteners—Beverages—"Doctor, Can I Cheat?"—Expect a Weight Loss—Being Flexible—Over-eating—Food Allergies—Vitamin and Mineral Supplements—Melvyn R. Werbach, M.D.—Out of Sight, Out of Mind—When Dining Out—Out of the Past—Cayce's discourse # 563-4—Author's Comments—Hippocrates, The Father of Medicine 73

tion—Backfire!—When two patients met—Recognizing "wrong" thinking—The Mental Formula of Emile Coué—Coué's "Secret"—The conscious and subconscious mind—Effective self-hypnosis—Coué's "String of Beads"—Troward's "The Hidden Power"—Practicing the Art of Visualization—The Alpha and the Omega—Release from Bondage by Imaging—Norman Vincent Peale on Imaging—William James, the Father of American Psychology—The Law of Expectancy

CHAPTER 11
The Crowning Glory

Psoriasis on the Scalp—Does Psoriasis Cause Hair Loss?—Psoriasis Along the Hairline—For Itchy Scalp—Shampoo Treatment for a Scaly-Psoriatic Scalp—Electric Heat-Cap/Oil Treatment

CHAPTER 12
Psoriasis on the Hands and Feet

Reasons for including this chapter—Effective measures—On Very Difficult Cases—When Washing Dishes—Two Stories of Success—Home Whirlpool Therapy—Fig. 12-1, Hands—Fig. 12-2, Feet—Patient: B.K.—Fig. 12-3, Fig. 12-4—Patient: L.M.—Fig. 12-5, Fig. 12-6—A Word of Caution—Summary—A Lesson in Patience—The value of having Patience and Persistence

CHAPTER 13
The Healing Process

First indications of success—Types of healing—A Very Special Case—The story of little L —Fig. 13-1—Fig. 13-2—Fig. 13-3—Fig. 13-4—Fig. 13-5—Fig. 13-6—The parents persist—A special gift from little L. Fig. 13-7

CHAPTER 14
Pushing the Panic Button

Alerting my patients—Two bothersome reactions—Family Reactions—When Prompt Attention is Necessary—Allergic Reactions—Avoiding Allergens

CHAPTER 15
The Arthritic Connection

Statistics—Types of psoriatic arthritis—About Arthritis—Virus Link?—Robert Simpson, M.D.—Same Problem/Different View—The value of maintaining alkalinity—Charles P.

ACKNOWLEDGMENTS

This volume was made possible by the kind and generous assistance of the following individuals and/or organizations. In their own way, they helped turn this dream into a reality.

• Joanne Richmond (dear friend and loyal secretary for many years) • Justine Skiba • Mildred and Frank DeLuca • Ingrid and Klaus A. Werner, • Barbara, Al and Steve Riecker • Leslie Del Rosso • Reva and Stanley I. Elkins • Elisabeth and Peter Henderson • Thea Wheelwright • Sharon Solomon • Marie Diehl • Sydne and Stephen Salmieri • Jerry Ruotolo • Howard Lockwood • Linda Cutrupi • Jonas Honig • Jean Munzer • Norbert Mester • Alice Gilmore (T.L.C.) • Charles Thomas Cayce, Jeanette Thomas, Judith Stevens Allison and All My Friends at The Association for Research and Enlightenment (A.R.E.) and The Edgar Cayce Foundation, Virginia Beach, VA •

and

To the patients themselves for their cooperation in allowing me to document and publish their personal case histories and photographs.

IN MEMORIAM

• My dear father, John J. Pagano, Esq. • Hugh Lynn Cayce • Gladys Davis Turner • Gina Cerminara • H. J. Reilly • Martha and Nick Nicklin • Judge Harold Gilmore • and my beloved, Shane

ILLUSTRATIONS AND PHOTOGRAPHS

Chapter 13 **The Healing Process**

Chapter 18 **The Emotional Factor**

COLOR PHOTOGRAPHIC PORTFOLIO

Patient: L.G. (Generalized Psoriasis)
   1. 2/17/83   2. 5/19/83   3. 6/5/85

Patient: J.C. (Common/Pustular)
   1. 4/6/84   2. 6/15/84   3. 9/5/84

Patient: J.R. (Common Vulgaris)
   1. 7/7/83   2. 11/10/83   3. 8/27/84

Patient: S.R. (Pustular Psoriasis)
   1. 6/10/80   2. 4/18/81   3. 2/12/85

Patient: A.M. (Generalized/Erythrodermic)
   1. 4/2/87   2. 5/5/87   3. 7/21/87

Patient: M.F. (Guttate)
   1. 3/1/86   2. 5/20/86   3. 7/11/86

Patient: T.O. (Generalized Psoriasis)
   1 & 3. 2/23/90   2 & 4. 4/28/90

BIBLIOGRAPHY

Allen, James, *As a Man Thinketh*, (Mt. Vernon, NY, Peter Pauper Press), pp. 9, 58-59.

Bach, Marcus, *The Chiropractic Story*, (Los Angeles, CA, De Vorss & Co., copyright 1968).

Best, Charles, M.D., and Norman Taylor, M.D., *The Living Body*, (New York, NY, Henry Holt & Co., copyright 1952, ed. 3), p. 381.

Best, Charles, M.D., and Norman Taylor, M.D., *The Physiological Basis of Medical Practice*, (Baltimore, The Williams & Wilkins Company, copyright 1955, ed. 6).

Bieler, Henry G., M.D., *Food is Your Best Medicine*, (New York, NY, copyright 1973, Random House, Inc.) pp 42-43.

Bloom, William, M.D. and Don W. Fawcett, M.D., *A Textbook of Histology*, (Philadelphia, London, Toronto, W.B. Saunders Company, copyright 1975, ed. 10) p. 659.

Bolduc, Henry Leo, *Self-Hypnosis, Creating Your Own Destiny*, (Virginia Beach, VA, A.R.E. Press, copyright 1985 by the Edgar Cayce Foundation).

Bourdillon, J.F., *Spinal Manipulation* (London, William Heinemann Medical Books Ltd. and Appleton-Century Crofts, New York, ed. 3, 1982). p. 2.

Brody, Jane E., "Emotions Found to Influence Nearly Every Human Ailment," *The New York Times*, (May 24, 1983) pp. C-1 & C-8.

Cayce, Edgar, *Readings*, (Virginia Beach, VA, The Edgar Cayce Foundation, copyright 1971), Reference 2455-2, Reference 2002-1, Reference 306-3, Reference 281-54.

Childers, Norman F., Ph.D., *Arthritis—Childers' Diet to Stop It*, (Gainesville, FL, Horticultural Publications, copyright 1977).

Circulating Files on Psoriasis, (Virginia Beach, VA, A.R.E. Press, copyright 1971 by the Edgar Cayce Foundation) Vols. 1 & 2.

Coué, Emile, *Self Mastery Through Conscious Autosuggestion*, (London WCIA, UNWIN HYMAN LTD., 40 Museum Street)

Davis, Adelle, *Let's Get Well*, (New York, NY, Harcourt, Brace & World, Inc. 1965) p. 156.

French's Index of Differential Diagnosis (Bristol, Publ. John Wright & Sons, Ltd. copyright 1954, ed. 7) Edited by Arthur H. Douthwaite, M.D.

Gauguelin, Michael, *How Atmospheric Conditions Affect Your Health*, (New York, NY, Stein and Day Publishers, 7 East 48th Street).

Gray, Henry F.R.S., *Gray's Anatomy*, (Philadelphia, Lea & Febiger, copyright 1954, ed. 26 by Goss).

Grossbart, Ted A., Ph.D., "Bringing Peace to Embattled Skin," *Psychology Today*, (Feb. 1982), p. 55, 59.

Hall, Manly P., *Healing, The Divine Art* (copyright 1943 by Manly Palmer Hall, Los Angeles, CA., pub. by the Philosophical Research Society, Inc.) pp. 238, 260, 261.

Houssay, Bernard A., M.D., *Human Physiology*, (New York, Toronto, London, McGraw-Hill Book Company, Inc., copyright 1951 and 1955, ed. 2).

Jensen, Bernard, D.C., Ph.D., and Sylvia Bell, *Tissue Cleansing Through Bowel Management*, (Escondido, CA, Bernard Jensen, D.C., copyright 1981, ed. 6).

Kleiner, Israel S., Ph.D., *Human Biochemistry*, (St. Louis, The C.V. Mosby Co., copyright 1954, ed. 4) p. 543.

Kloss, Jethro, *Back to Eden*, (New York, NY, pub. Laurer Books, Inc., copyright 1971), pp. 212-213.

Lansford, Frederick D., M.D., "Commentary on Psoriasis" in *Physician's Reference Notebook*, ed. by William A. McGarey, M.D., (Virginia Beach, VA, The A.R.E. P{ress, Sept. 1968., Ed.1) p. 189—Extracted from References 5016-1 and 622-1.

Lewis, George M., M.D., *Practical Dermatology* (Philadelphia & London, W. B. Saunders Company, copyright 1952).

Lowe, Nicholas J., M.D., "Systemic Treatment of Severe Psoriasis—The Role of Cyclosporine," *The New England Journal of Medicine*, January 31, 1991 (Vol. 324, No. 5 copyright 1991, by the Massachusetts Medical Society) pp. 333-334.

Lucas, Richard, *Secrets of the Chinese Herbalists*, (West Nyack, NY, pub. Parker Publishing Co., Inc., copyright 1977), pp. 191-192.

Marks, Dr. Ronald, *Psoriasis*, (New York, NY, Arco Publishing, Inc., copyright 1981, p. 32.)

Maximow, Alexander A. and William Bloom, *A Textbook of Histology*, (Philadelphia and London, W. B. Saunders Company, copyright 1952, ed. 6).

McGarey, William A., M.D., "Rheumatoid Arthritis", *Pathways to Health* (June/July 1979, Medical Research Bulletin. Volume 1, No. 2., The A.R.E. Clinic, Inc., Phoenix, AZ).

McGarey, William A., M.D., Article "Indigestion," *Health Care Report* (Vol. 1, No. 4, pub. The Edgar Cayce Foundation, Virginia Beach, VA).

McGarey, William A., M.D., "Olive Oil May Protect the Heart", *Pathways to Health* (Phoenix, AZ, The A.R.E. Clinic, Inc., Vol. 7, No. 3).

Monroe, Anne Shannon, *Singing In The Rain*, (Garden City, NY, pub. The Sun Dial Press, copyright 1926 by Doubleday, Doran & Co.) p. 206

"More than one way to skin a chicken"—*Tufts University Diet and Nutrition Letter* (Food for Thought—Vol. 8, No. 10, December 1990) p. 7.

Pathogenesis of Visceral Disease Following Vertebral Lesions (Chicago, IL, pub. by the American Osteopathic Association, 1948) p. 232.

Pottenger, Francis M., M.D., *Symptoms of Visceral Disease*, ed. 7, (St. Louis, 1953, The C.V. Mosby Co.) p. 9, 42, 135, 144, 272, 280, 410.

Psoriasis, Washington, D.C., DHEW Publication No. (NIH) 77-1104, U.S. Government Printing Office, 1977.

Reilly, Harold J. and Ruth Hagy Brod, *The Edgar Cayce Handbook for Health Through Drugless Therapy* (New York, NY, Macmillan Publishing Co., Inc. copyright 1975, ed. 1).

Scott, Eugene J., M.D., and Eugene M. Farber, M.D., *Dermatology in General Medicine* (New York, NY, 1971, McGraw-Hill Inc.) Chapter 8—p. 226.

"Shucking the Myth About Cholesterol in Shellfish"—*Tufts University Diet and Nutrition Letter* (Food for Thought Vol 5, No. 4, June 1987) p. 7.

Sugrue, Thomas, *There Is A River*, (New York, Chicago, San Francisco. Holt, Rinehart and Winston Publishers, copyright 1942 & 1945, revised edition).

Troward, Thomas, *The Edinburgh Lectures on Mental Science*, (New York, NY, Dodd, Mead & Company, copyright 1909) pp. 84-85.

Troward, Thomas, *The Hidden Power*, (New York, NY, Dodd, Mead & Company, copyright 1921 by S.A. Troward, 1961 by Dodd, Mead & Company) pp 97-98.

Wachhorst, Wyn, *Thomas Alva Edison—An American Myth*, (Cambridge, MA, and London, England, The MIT Press, copyright 1981).

Werback, Melvyn R., M.D., *Nutritional Influence on Illness*, (New Canaan, CN, Keats Publishing, Inc., copyright 1987-1988) pg. 372.

Wolberg, Lewis, R.M.D., *Medical Hypnosis* (New York, NY, Grune & Stratton, copyright 1948).

Zinsser, William, *On Writing Well*, (New York, NY, pub. Harper & Row, copyright 1976), p. 55.